The Internet for Orthopaedists

Springer
New York
Berlin
Heidelberg
Hong Kong
London
Milan
Paris
Tokyo

THE
INTERNET
FOR
ORTHOPAEDISTS

With 56 Illustrations

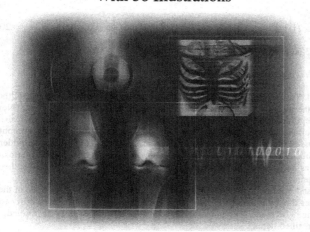

DON JOHNSON, M.D.
Carleton University
and University of Ottawa
Ottawa, Ontario
Canada

MYLES CLOUGH, M.D.
University of British Columbia
Vancouver, British Columbia
and
Royal Inland Hospital
Kamloops, British Columbia
Canada

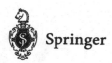
Springer

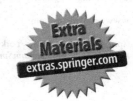
Extra
Materials
extras.springer.com

Don Johnson, M.D.
Sports Medicine Clinic,
Carleton University
and
Orthopaedic Surgery,
University of Ottawa
Ottawa, Ontario K1S B56
Canada
donnie@igs.net

Myles Clough, M.D.
Department of Orthopaedics,
University of British Columbia
British Columbia V2C 6G6
and
Royal Inland Hospital
Kamloops, British Columbia
Canada
mylesclough@shaw.ca

Library of Congress Cataloging-in-Publication Data
Johnson, Donald.
    The Internet for orthopaedists/Donald Johnson, Myles Clough.
        p. cm.
    Includes bibliographical references and index.
    Additional material to this book can be downloaded from http://extra.springer.com.
    ISBN 0-387-95483-X (softcover : alk. paper)
        1. Orthopedics.   2. Orthopedists.   3. Medicine—Computer network resources.   4. Internet.
    I. Title.
    RD732.J585 2002
    025.06'6167—dc21   2002020942

ISBN 0-387-95483-X   Printed on acid-free paper.

Printed in the United States of America.

9 8 7 6 5 4 3 2 1   SPIN 10874736

Typesetting: Pages created by Matrix Publishing Services, York, PA.

www.springer-ny.com

Springer-Verlag   New York Berlin Heidelberg
A member of BertelsmannSpringer Science+Business Media GmbH

Series Preface

The Internet is the ultimate amalgamation of the Information Age and the Communication Age. It is a technology that took 40 years to become an overnight sensation, moving from the province of computer geeks to household utility in short order, once it was discovered. We have gone from thinking a URL was a form of alien presence to viewing it as a natural footnote to bus advertising.

Like the Internet itself, interest in computing, both local and distant, has grown exponentially. Now grandmothers send e-mails to their stockbrokers, meals are planned and the groceries purchased across the Web, and music videos can be previewed or concert tickets purchased—all with the help of the Internet. When our children come home from school, they are as likely to sign on to the Internet as they are to turn on the television. The Internet is a universal commodity, for those with access.

The American Internet User Survey found that more than 41.5 million adults in the United States actively are using the Internet. Of these Web users, 51% use the Web on a daily basis. It seems everybody needs to be connected to the Web, just as they all seem to need to make cell-phone calls while changing lanes in heavy traffic. The Internet is nothing less than a library card to the world. At the most basic level, the Internet is a high-speed web of worldwide computer-based information resources. It is a network of computer networks. One moment you can be browsing through the Library of Congress or looking at pictures from the National Library of Medicine, and the next moment conversing with a colleague in Indonesia.

What about the Internet and medicine? Well, we, physicians, sell information. That is what we do in medicine. That is what we always have done. Today, the difference is that we do it in an age built on information. Information, medical and otherwise, is all around us. From pocket pagers that deliver stock quotes and sports scores to palm-top digital assistance that wirelessly connects to the Internet, information is achieving the status of Oxygen†—it is all around us and invisible. Today, informa-

---

†Oxygen also is the name of a computing project at the Massachusetts Institute of Technology that is aimed at achieving this goal.

tion is managed, moved, and organized in ways never thought of in the past and will soon be managed in ways not yet conceived. In medicine, information is vital, but the exponential growth of knowledge available requires new approaches to its dissemination, access, and use. Central to this is the Internet. Information is now the province of anyone with a computer. This has led to "disintermediation": the ability of consumers to go directly to the source of information (or goods and services), bypassing the intermediate steps of providers. In medicine, this means that physicians obtain and distribute information in new ways, patients obtain and receive their information in new ways, and, together, patients and providers interact in new ways. Very little has remained the same, yet, fundamentally, nothing is different—we still sell information. Medicine has frequently led the way with new technology: We used print materials when books were in their infancy; we embraced the telephone like few other professions; pagers, two-way radio, and teleconferencing (telemedicine) were all adopted by medicine early in their development. The need for information always has driven this adoption, and it is no different for the Internet.

This series of texts on the Internet in medicine and in medical subspecialty areas hopes to assist in this natural evolution in two ways. First, it will help us understand the abilities of the Internet and know its tools so that we may capitalize on what the Internet holds for ourselves as physicians and our patients. Second, the medical applications of the Internet have grown too rapidly and are too specialty-specific to explore in depth in any single volume. Hence, the birth of specialty-specific volumes. When the first edition of *The Internet for Physicians* was published, it was mainly the technophile fringe that was surfing. The first edition attempted to introduce the concept of information transfer and communication and point the way toward a tool of the future. The second edition attempted to assuage trepidation in the use of this emerging tool and suggest the why and wherefore of being connected. The needs that drove those goals almost have completely disappeared. The third edition is more focused on the medical aspects of the Internet and its use, and much less on the nuts and bolts of connecting and communicating through the Web. This evolution has opened the possibility of a series dedicated to the Internet in various specialties of medicine. Each of these volumes deals with specialty-specific aspects of the Internet, going beyond the general scope of *The Internet for Physicians*. Each author has been chosen for his or her expertise in medical computing, and they are each a recognized leader in their field. Each volume builds on fundamentals introduced in *The Internet for Physicians*. While each volume stands alone, they have all been created so that each fits within the same concept. As authors, we hope that this series will open new and exciting options for this new age of medical information. Surf's up!

Roger P. Smith, M.D.
University of Missouri–Kansas City School of Medicine
Kansas City, Missouri, USA
Author of *The Internet for Physicians*

Preface

A book about using the Orthopaedic Internet has two potential groups of readers: those who already use the Internet for orthopaedic information and those who don't but are considering it. Although there is some overlap between the needs of these two groups, it would be difficult to satisfy everyone and there is a danger of being too superficial for one group and too detailed for the other. We have tried to use the inherent difference between the two groups to solve this problem. For the group that is not familiar with the Internet and computerized information technology (IT), the printed text is an introduction to the Internet with leads to the immense resources on the Net itself. For this group the CD-ROM has a list of links to the resources discussed in the text. We have also prepared a Web site with basic workshops and tutorials on finding orthopaedic information and straightforward ways to improve use of the basic IT programs. For experienced readers, we believe that the book alone will not be enough and that they will want to interact with the material and look up the Internet resources referred to as they go. For this group we have posted a hypertext version so they can read and surf (http://condor.sechrest.com/clough/book/default.htm). The intended result is that the book is an overview dealing with the subjects to a certain level of sophistication. For more detail and for activities that involve connection to the Internet we recommend using the Web site. Since one of the main messages of this book is that IT provides a richer, deeper, and more personalized learning experience than text alone, it would be hypocrisy not to attempt to demonstrate that.

Many of the terms used in this book are unfamiliar or have unfamiliar meanings. There is an extensive glossary where the terms are further defined. Another difficult issue is acronyms. We cannot avoid using them. The term is written out in full when encountered for the first time in each chapter with the acronym in parentheses. All IT acronyms are glossary terms. You are on your own with orthopaedic ones although we do link to the Orthopaedic Acronym Finder on the CD-ROM.

Contents

1
The Basics

Introduction

Just in case you haven't noticed, the Internet is a revolution in communication and commerce that will rival the other great media revolutions of the past such as radio and television. Depending upon your viewpoint, it may rank up there with the industrial revolution or the invention of printing for the degree of change that it will make in our lives, or due to its lurid content, it may simply be the instrument of the devil. It is impossible to predict just how this will unfold in the next few years, but if the past decade is any indication, it will be fast-paced and exciting. There will be a few setbacks, such as the recent dot-com fiasco and wrong directions taken, but the end result is going to change the way we communicate, teach, learn, buy, bank, book our travel, search for medical information, and so on. The Internet is a complex topic, and we have learned a lot while researching and writing about the subject. How much of this do you have to know? For most of your daily use of the Internet, you only have to know how to connect, open your e-mail, or click on a hyperlink to open a site on the World Wide Web. This reference material is provided for that time when you may be interested in finding out more detail about the Internet. Just how did this whole thing start?

History of the Internet

The Internet is a collection of millions of computers connected together to share information. The complexity of the network is what makes the Internet intriguing. The Internet originated in 1969 as a military project designed to reliably link remote computers together using phone lines. University researchers saw the benefit of joining computers together and got on board. This led to the development of TCP/IP (Transmission Control Protocol/Internet Protocol). The browser breaks the information down according to the TCP protocol into small packets that are sent through routers over many intermediate computers. When they arrive at the destination address, the browser reassembles the message according to the IP protocol.

The Internet remained the domain of the elite at universities into the 1990s. In 1993, the World Wide Web (WWW) was developed, browser programs were written to locate the many pages of linked information, and the Internet exploded. Hypertext markup language (html) was developed to show text, images, and graphics on the same page. The Web browser (originally Mosaic, later Netscape, and much later Internet Explorer) allowed the user to view these pages without any special technical knowledge. This paved the way for the use of the Internet by the average person with a phone line, a modem, and a computer. In those early years it was difficult to configure the connection, and expert technical help was often required. Now the computer is completely set up by the supplier, and only a few mouse clicks and your credit card are required to connect to the Internet.

The financial support for the Internet comes from government, commercial advertising, and the user. Government funds the local networks that connect the government agencies. Universities support their own high-speed connections. Local service providers saw the opportunity to charge a fee to connect the local user to the Internet. Large organizations such as AOL (American Online), MSN (Microsoft Networks), and Prodigy became the key players in providing an easy way to connect to the Internet by supplying a portal with e-mail, a browser to view Web pages, and chat rooms to communicate with other users. These large commercial services joined with other media giants, for example, AOL Time Warner, to become the major players in providing access to the Internet. These services then became the portals of entry to the Internet with e-mail, chat groups, messaging services, and, of course, advertising aimed at the client. In the spirit of the Internet, the freenet services have survived, and most communities have a free connection to the Internet supported by volunteers and user donations. For example, the Ottawa freenet is administered from Carleton University. You need to have a connection to the Internet via an ISP (Internet service provider), which may be the "free" always-on connection via the university or hospital, or through a dialup modem. The site offers information about schools, community activities, libraries, and special interest groups. To connect to the Ottawa freenet, go to a search engine and type "Ottawa freenet." A choice will appear; click on "National capital freenet," and the page **http://www.galaxy.com/hytelnet/ FRE017.html** will connect you to the local information. This gives you the "feel" of a community. You can find out what is happening in town without leaving your computer chair. The freenet also offers text-only e-mail that many retro people find appealing.

There is a gradual realization that with declining ad revenues, there will have to be a charge for some of the content. *The Wall Street Journal* charges a user fee for its Web site archives. This is a niche market that, in a business, may be written off as expenses, but it also may signify one of the major changes for the future of the Internet. If you manage a Web site with information only, with no product to sell, another model of financing this business must be entertained. This is an evolving concept that challenges the original idea that the Internet is free for all. Many orthopaedic journals have full-text versions of their articles available free to subscribers or as pay-per-view (PPV)

Information and Information Technology

How Is the Information Stored and Transferred?

The information is stored in millions of different computers around the world. These are linked through an extensive network controlled by routers. You can connect computer to computer via Telnet or by File Transfer Protocol (FTP). Any connection to the Internet allows access to your computer by anyone who wants to enter and be malicious. The solution is to designate certain computers as servers and store files on that server for anyone to view. These outside computers are separated from your main network of information by a firewall. Telnet and FTP both require that you know a specific address to connect to the other computer and usually a password, giving a minor degree of security to the connection.

The basic Internet connection consists of four parts: the user's desktop called the client computer, the Internet service provider (ISP), the host computer (file server) where the information is stored for you to access, and finally the network that links all this together. The user starts his computer and opens his connection to the Internet, which may be via dialup modem, always on cable, broadband DSL (digital subscriber line), or satellite connection. The client now has a connection to the Internet through an Internet service provider. Any program running on the client computer that needs information from the Internet sends a message to the ISP giving the Internet address of the resource the user wants. The ISP in turn then routes a message through the network to request the files from the host computer. The host computer then sends the files (using TCP/IP) to the ISP which passes them on to the client computer ready for use by the program that originally made the request. The client may use an e-mail program to send and receive e-mail messages, open a browser, such as Internet Explorer, and view Web pages or connect to chat rooms or instant messaging programs to communicate with friends.

There are alternatives to the basic modem connection. If you are located in a large organization, you can use a LAN (local area network) to connect directly to the Internet without the use of a modem. The organization may have a high-speed connection and allow all employees to connect to the Internet using a router. If you are a broadband phone subscriber, you may use a router to send the always-on connection to your local area network. The advantage of the router is that it acts as a firewall to prevent someone from hacking into your open system. The cable television companies also provide this always-on high-speed connection through a router.

In order to connect to Web pages your browser program has to know the address of the page that you want to view. This address is called a URL, uniform resource locator. A typical URL for the Arthroscopy Association is **http://www.aana.org**. The http stands for hypertext transfer protocol and indicates a hypertext page that is found on the World Wide Web. The address of the association is aana.org. The suffix ".org" denotes that the domain belongs to an organization, usually a nonprofit one. It is one of the several domain suffixes, such as .com, .edu, .mil, and the like. Often another suffix will indicate the country where the server is located, such as .ca for Canada. So the frequently used phrase "dot-com" refers to an organization with a ".com" suffix to its URL indicating that it is a commercial enterprise. By extension the term "dot-com enterprise" is often used for organizations that conduct most of their business through the Internet and have very little substance in the real world.

The information is sent in small packets of information that are routed around the networks to the destination address. The routers are hardware devices with input and output ports. The routers read the address information as it comes in, and redirect it to another router closer to the destination address. This address is a series of four block numbers, such as "219.112.221.255." The number obviously makes sense to a computer, but it is difficult for us to remember what the number refers to, and so the URL is the text to which the number is assigned. For instance, the above number may be assigned to the Internet domain name of **http://www.aana.org**.

The other prefix that is commonly used is"ftp://" for file transfer protocol. You may also see the prefix "mailto" before the e-mail address, such as **mailto: joeblow@home.com**. This denotes the type of file that is being transferred. Now most of the browsers allow you to shorten the entry to **www.aana.org** from **http://www.aana.org**, but in the browser address window, the full name will be displayed. Because of the integration between the WINDOWS™ operating system (OS) and the Internet Explorer browser you can type the URL, for example, "owl.orthogate.com," in any address window and your computer will recognize this as an Internet address, connect to the Internet, and deliver the page.

Whereas human brains usually make no distinction between information in upper- and lowercase text, computers make an important distinction between them. URLs are all case sensitive, so be careful to use exactly the correct case. In general the Internet likes lowercase text addresses.

A central registry at **www.register.com** registers all the domain names. You can go to the site, enter a name, and see if it has been previously registered. If not, for a fee, you can then register the name. If the original name **www.aana.org** is taken, then **www.aana.com** may be available and can be registered. The common domain suffixes are as follows:

.com—commercial	**.gov**—government
.org—nonprofit organizations	**.mil**—military
.edu—educational	**.net**—nonprofit organizations

There is now a rush to purchase the new release of domain names on speculation that someone will come along and offer the owner a million dollars for the brand name: .tv or .bus.

There are also geographical domain suffixes.

.at—Austria	**.gr**—Greece
.au—Australia	**.no**—Norway
.be—Belgium	**.jp**—Japan
.ca—Canada	**.sw**—Sweden
.ch—Switzerland	**.uk**—United Kingdom (Britain)
.de—Germany	**.us**—United States
.fr—France	

Most of the documents stored on the Internet are written in Hypertext Markup Language or .html, frequently abbreviated to .htm. When searching for a file this suffix must be attached. An example of this is **http://www.medmedia.com/ooa1/52.htm**. When this is typed a Web page will appear from the Web site of *Wheeless' Textbook* on pilon fractures. The address **http://www.medmedia.com/ooa1/52** without the .htm will not be accepted and you will get the dreaded error 404, "The page cannot be found."

There are other suffixes that are used to denote file types:

.html–Hypertext Markup Language
.index–the main page of a Web site
.txt–plain-text document
.jpeg or .gif–a picture or graphics file
.zip–a compressed file in WINDOWS™
.sit–a Macintosh compressed file, and
.doc–a Microsoft Word (word processor) document, usually only seen in
    attachments to e-mail.

E-mail addresses generally relate to the same domain address. For example, a Web site is **http://www.sportsmed.com** and an e-mail address for this site is **anybody@sportsmed.com**

There are several common file types used on the Internet. The ASCII (American Standard Code for Information Interchange) text files are used for text e-mail messages. These files have no formatting and can be read by any computer and all software programs. You should set your e-mail program to use plain-text files to allow everyone to view your messages.

Adobe Acrobat PDF is an executable program that interprets and displays its own format, PDF (portable document format), requiring a special reader to view these files. (The download is free, at **www.adobe.com.**) The advantage of the PDF files is that they can be viewed on both PC and Mac computers. Unlike HTML files they also print out in a "what you see is what you get" (WYSIWYG) fashion. This format is extensively used to convert documents that were designed for paper into computer files.

One other type of file used on the Internet is the compressed file ".zip" for the WINDOWS™ file compression (winzip at **www.winzip.com**) and the ".sit" files from Macintosh. Both of these file types require special software to compress and uncompress the files at both ends of the transmission. The advantages of this type of file are both the compression into a smaller file, and all the information being sent in one packet.

Information Technology

In addition to providing a guide for orthopaedic surgeons newly arrived on the Internet, this book makes several fundamental points. The first is that the existence of the Internet will make changes in every facet of orthopaedic communication, among surgeons, between teachers and trainees, between surgeons and patients, and between the medical profession and the public. Those changes will be as sweeping and have as large an impact as the invention of printing. They will happen whether we want them or not, whether we understand them or not, and whether we are ready for them or not. The second point is that orthopaedic surgeons are being deluged with information and that electronic information technology offers one of the few viable solutions to this problem. The third point is that any solution to the problems of overload and any rational response to the challenges of the Internet require an official clearinghouse for orthopaedic information. We believe that cooperating to establish such a clearinghouse should be an urgent priority for all the official orthopaedic organizations of the world.

We refer frequently in this book to the "Orthopaedic Internet" and we may be challenged that no such entity exists. The Orthopaedic Internet exists on many levels: as the collection of orthopaedic sites, many of which interlink with one another; as the community of orthopaedists who are interested in the use of the Internet to promote and teach orthopaedics; and as the vast, chaotic, tangled web of sites from patients, suppliers, information merchants, and snake oil salesmen that offer orthopaedic advice and information. We need to ensure that the voice of scientific orthopaedics is heard clearly on the Internet. So, if you feel that there is no "Orthopaedic Internet," you should join with us to create it!

Innovation

If you look back over the last twenty years in orthopaedic surgery, it would be difficult to find a single operation that is done in exactly the same way or for exactly the same indications. All these innovations have come to our attention as improvements, but so have thousands of other ideas that have been rejected or have never caught on. It would be gratifying if this discrimination were the result of meticulous use of scientific orthopaedic information but we all know that commercial pressures, the flavor of the moment, and the excitement of trying new things have a part to play as well. Indeed, there have been innovations, such as pes anserinus transfer or metal-backed patella resurfacing, that have been widely adopted but which turned out poorly. So we can view the past and the future as a continuum of innovation beset with traps and blind alleys. Each of us must take an individual path through this maze trying to give our patients the benefit of a forward-looking innovative practice balanced by caution and a healthy skepticism. The aggregated choices of all of us create "progress" in orthopaedics, and even then, some of the activity will actually be misdirected.

The standard path through the maze is to make changes based on the best available scientific information. The trouble arises in construing the terms "best," "available," and "scientific information." In the context of our present discussion access to scientific information is the most critical issue. It is likely true that the answer to most of our information needs is down on paper somewhere. Finding out where and finding the piece of paper in time is a huge challenge. The traditional way to come up with the best available scientific evidence is to "keep up with the literature." This can be taken to mean randomly reading the orthopaedic journals and changing your management strategies and thought processes to accommodate the new information. Some people maintain a card index with references to papers they have read but most rely on memory and their amazing ability to associate and subconsciously organize information. There is no question that the most valuable piece of information technology hardware is still the human brain (wetware!).

Under the paradigm of "keeping up" you don't just read what you need, you read everything so that when you need it you have it. In the MEDLINE database of medical literature maintained by the US National Library of Medicine there are 102 journals whose main subject is orthopaedics, orthopaedic sports medicine, arthroscopy, or hand surgery. There are more journals whose primary focus is biomechanics, biophysics, rheumatology, rehabilitation medicine, neurosurgery, and surgery in general. There are yet more on other subjects of interest to orthopaedists, such as artificial limbs, radiology, aging, osteoporosis, pain, orthopaedic nursing, physiotherapy, hand therapy, podiatry, chiropractic, injury prevention, and so on. To keep up with the orthopaedic literature would mean that an orthopaedic surgeon with general interests would have to read or be aware of the contents of all 102 journals. Assuming an average of 8 issues a year and 25 articles per issue, one arrives at more than 20,000 articles a year to internalize in order to do this. To continue the *argumentum ad absurdum* we may assume that you can skim the contents of each article in five minutes and do not have to spend time obtaining the journals in question. Sitting at your conveyor belt and reading orthopaedics full time, 24 hours a day, it would take you nearly 70 days each year to complete your task of keeping up with the orthopaedic literature!

So those who claim to keep up with the orthopaedic literature obviously must be doing some selection and discarding as unworthy of their attention a huge proportion of the world's scientific orthopaedic effort. Even if you only read reviews, the coverage of current orthopaedic issues would be full of holes. Of course, this is not the only thing that people do. When faced with a specific problem they will "go to the books," "do a literature search," or in some fashion conduct a "just-in-time" review of the orthopaedic literature available to them. Our fundamental argument is that this focused review of orthopaedic information, as and when you need it, is made far more feasible by electronic information technology and is a more valuable use of time than the random "keeping up" process. It requires new skills. We should learn them and teach them.

Wise choices derive from a synthesis of experience and the best available information. Information, in turn, is organized data. Although information is data transformed in some way, it is as well to remember the transformation is done with a purpose and that most information is slanted.

Information

If the gathering of data is the bedrock of science, the transformation of data into information has many layers. Typically in a scientific publication the first layer will involve mathematical manipulations to obtain sums or means. The next may be to perform statistical calculations to determine the significance of differences between aggregated observations. The next may be to compare the new findings with others reported previously. Examples of the first level of transformation of data into information are given in Table 1.1.

As soon as the transformation occurs some of the information is lost. When we see an average range of motion there is no way of telling if some of the participants in the study had wildly aberrant values that skewed the result. Without the original data one cannot even tell if the values were distributed normally or perhaps in a bimodal distribution. If our reason for reading the article is reasonably casual, this doesn't matter. In fact we expect the authors to summarize their data so that we don't have to. We must be aware, however, that transforming data nearly al-

TABLE 1.1. Examples of data observations and the information derived from their transformation.

Observation	Transformation
X-ray image	Image with caption identifying the features of interest
Range of motion	Average range of motion for the study cohort
Pain description	Functional score

ways conceals the extent of variation and may introduce bias. It is a convenience based on the limitations of paper that we take these transformations on trust and this is one of the many things that the Internet may change. If we fully use the resources of cyberspace, the data, the calculations, and the foundations of what is reported could all be scrutinized and the trust we have in the authors' transformations and conclusions can be confirmed.

Information Technology (IT)

Virtually everyone uses information technology. Those who distrust and dislike using computers still have notebooks, ledgers, card files, and collections of reprints. Indeed, at the furthest remove, printing, writing, and even language can be considered information technology. Anything that has been invented to improve communication is information technology. We only tend to focus on computers because they are the newest element and perhaps because they have not been fully integrated into standard orthopaedic operating practice. It may be helpful to consider the paper-based information technology with which we are so familiar. You may not think of your photo album or a bookshelf as examples of information technology but they are indeed so.

Table 1.2 emphasizes that the electronic analog of paper IT is often much simpler in concept. Thus we can compress the entire cascade of

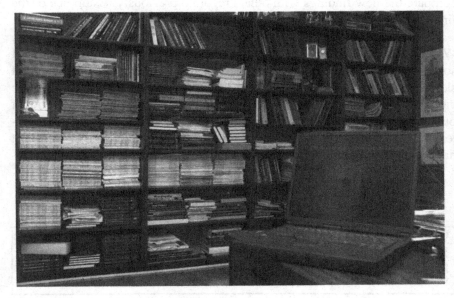

FIGURE 1.1. Information technology, both old and new, have their place

TABLE 1.2. Paper information technology with its electronic analog.

Paper technology	Purpose	Electronic analog
Notes	Information to be saved for future reference	Text file Word processor file
Notebook	Convenient way of making notes and keeping them together	Folder
File	Receptacle for related notes	Folder
File cabinet	Place to store and organize related files	Folder Disk
File room	Storage area for file cabinets	Folder Backup disk
Spreadsheet	Notebook with columns for related scientific or financial information	Spreadsheet file
Ledger	Spreadsheet of financial information	Spreadsheet Database file
Duplicate information	Copied information stored separately for convenience or to avoid loss	File copy
Photostat copy		Backup disk Mirror site
X-ray	Film with medical image	X-ray image file
X-ray packet	Envelope for storing related images, usually of one patient	Folder
Photograph	Print or film image	Image file
Album/slide tray	Collection of photographs	Folder
Article	Text, illustrations, and bibliography relating to a certain subject or research project	File Folder Web site
Book	Sequenced information in text or image form	Folder Web site
Bookshelf	Collection of books, often in random order	Folder
Library	Collection of books, usually indexed for easier retrieval	Folder CD-ROM Web site The Internet
Bibliography	Collection of citations related to a specific subject	MEDLINE URL File
Indexus Medicus	Annual publication summarizing medical publications	MEDLINE Search engine Index site
Citations index	List of papers cited in scientific publications	Search engine

file, file cabinet, file room, books, bookshelf, and library into one concept (folder) in electronic IT.

The details of electronic IT may be abstruse and beyond the comprehension of anyone without education in computer science, but the concepts are simple and require no special training. Anyone who can organize an office or a household can design and implement a file and folder structure that would allow them to store and retrieve orthopaedic information in all its complexity and variety.

It is even correct to say that there are very few electronic procedures that do not have a paper analog. One might think that searching and indexing large databases are only possible with computer help but this is not true. It was possible to trace a telephone call in the days before computers. One could either set a team to read through the telephone directory to find the required number and hence its address, or use a list indexed by number as the telephone company and law enforcement agencies would do. It wasn't impossible, just time-consuming, boring, difficult, or restricted.

We hope to ease the transition from a solely paper form of IT to a combination. It's highly unlikely that many people will make a transition exclusively to electronic IT. Although the scribbled note and the individual patient file could be eliminated with personal digital assistants (PDAs), notes are familiar and (fairly) convenient. People will choose their own mix of paper and electronic IT.

Advantages of Electronic IT Over Paper

It has been suggested that computers have never saved any money or eliminated work or workers; all that has happened is that we can do things that couldn't be done before without enormous effort. It is also easy to adduce the advertising pressure and the power of fashion to explain why computers are "taking over." When you factor in the frustrations of system crashes, the need to keep upgrading, virus exposure, and the anxiety induced by constantly having to learn new procedures, it may be far from clear why we should make any effort in the direction of electronic IT. But the phenomenal growth in computer applications is based now on widespread adoption throughout the economy and throughout teaching and health care institutions. Unless all these people are being bamboozled there must be some advantages.

Correctable

Many people's first exposure to electronic IT is to word-processing programs. The overwhelming selling point is that if you make an error, you don't have to retype the whole document or mess around with "white-out." The whole process of editing or rearranging a document is much easier and this may make it more likely that a document is reworked thoroughly before it is "finished." Whether this results in better documents overall is debatable but would anyone prefer to go back to the typewriter or to manuscript?

Fast

Computer operations are amazingly fast. In fact, if there is a detectable interval between our actions and the computer's response, we wonder if there isn't a glitch. In practical terms the speed of operation allows us to program computers to perform multiple repetitive tasks such as searching. Enormous amounts of data and information can be sent over computer networks in a very short time.

Accurate

Because of the binary nature of computer operations they are highly reproducible in a properly coded program. This translates into superhuman accuracy in operations such as calculations and comparisons. Searching is one operation that takes full advantage of the speed and accuracy of computer operations. Large volumes of data can be searched for a particular word or number and the result is reliable. As we have noted earlier this is not truly a qualitative difference between paper and electronic systems. Both are searchable in theory. However, the advantage in speed and accuracy in an electronic system is so pronounced that the difference is almost a qualitative one. Certainly, we incorporate searching strategies using electronic IT in a way we would never do in a paper system. Because databases such as MEDLINE are searchable in seconds it is now reasonable to recommend just-in-time updates to your knowledge as opposed to trying to keep up in every field. Of course, computer operations go wrong, crash, or produce nonsensical results. This is only rarely the result of hardware glitches. Most often the programmer or the user—fallible humans—has failed to take advantage of the computer's accuracy.

Undegradable

Because the numbers in electronic files are binary and can be copied accurately they do not lose information. There is no fading or smudging. When one considers how many computers an image passed over the Internet may have been through, it is astonishing that the image we see is exactly the same as the image that was sent. As long as computers are connected to the Internet and are using the same protocols to communicate with one another the files are preserved unchanged. There may be concerns about hardware compatibility but as long as you can access a file over the network it will remain functionally intact.

Storage and Retrieval

In most programs storage and retrieval of documents and files is fast, simple, and foolproof. Although finding documents does require a system and a way of naming files that assists in the task, it can be made a lot easier and more intuitive than finding paper files in a cabinet.

Copying

A valuable consequence of the speed and accuracy of computer operations is that files can be copied rapidly, easily, and with complete accuracy. This makes backing up the information for safety a lot more manageable than a paper system. The backed-up version can be stored in a place geographically distant from the main institution to reduce the risk that a local disaster will destroy all records. Another advantage of accurate rapid copying is that sharing and distributing files is easy. This is one essential feature of the Internet.

Encryption

The technology of public key/private key encryption is another example of a process that could be done by hand but was so laborious that it was almost restricted to espionage. However, it is now incorporated into many routine electronic transactions and the conversion is so fast that we don't even recognize it is taking place. When you see a message that the connection with an Internet site is "secure," what is happening is that the two-way communication between the site and your computer is encrypted so that all the data being transmitted would be meaningless if intercepted. Only the computers at either end of the transaction know the encryption keys that are needed to translate the message "in clear." It is possible to encrypt all stored personal computer files. The security thus obtained is an order of magnitude better than anything obtainable through a paper system.

Updating

A consequence of computer files being rapidly and accurately correctable is that a communication need never be finalized. We know that new information is going to be produced shortly, which will affect the conclusions and interpretations in a document just published. Rewriting and republishing the work to incorporate this additional information is so labor intensive that it is very rarely done. One occasionally sees retractions in the literature and some articles stimulate a discussion on the correspondence pages but these are not incorporated into the original article. This is potentially dangerous, and electronic IT with its ready ability to update a document is superior in this regard. As our institutions mature in the use of electronic IT, updating should become integrated into the process of publication.

Text Versus Hypertext

A hypertext document contains links to other documents or files. The closest analogy to the paper system would be footnotes or the notation, "see map page 34." In general, text documents are rigidly structured with a beginning and an end. The author anticipates that the reader will begin at the beginning and read all the way through and designs the communication accordingly. Hypertext allows this linearity to remain but doesn't make it mandatory. If the total site is broken up into documents linked as hypertext, then readers can take individual paths through the information, reading and following links as they think best. In a text document the authors control what you read. In a hypertext document they offer you a menu.

We currently present our scholarship in a linear fashion with set order and content. Hypertext publications should change to a layered pattern and include a layman's version identifying the significance of this work in the real world. Authors will need to make adaptations to hypertext to get the greatest advantage from the medium. On the Web site (**http:// condor.sechrest.com/clough/book/default.htm**) we offer a summary of this book with links to all the different sections. This is to exemplify the difference between text and hypertext. It must be experienced, just as the difference between an illuminated manuscript scroll and a printed book needed to be experienced at the dawn of the Renaissance.

The Internet

Thus far we have been examining IT systems in isolation, but, of course, the existence of the Internet makes an enormous difference. The Internet started as a military and then an academic information exchange network. Despite the apparent takeover by commercial interests, it still functions extremely well in its original capacity. Predictions that the Internet will transform academic communication are thick on the ground. The main uncertainty seems to be how this will occur and what it will be!

What are the attributes that will drive these changes?

Speed

Not only is file transfer rapid, but the process of posting pages on the Internet is extremely rapid compared to all previous forms of publication. In the paper IT system the process of submitting a piece of scholarship, having it edited and reviewed, then having the printing set up and the eventual publication distributed could take months or years. On the Internet it would take only minutes to transform a document into a Web page and post it. If one paid a lot of attention to issues of style and presentation, it might take a week. In essence all the time is taken up in preparation, editing, and reviewing the work; publication and distribution take no time.

Economy

Publishing and distribution are the major costs of academic journals. Typically the authors, illustrators, reviewers, and even the editors are not paid directly by the journal. All the content valued by the readers is provided for free and the lion's share of the expense of books and journals to the reader is for publishing and distribution, the things the Internet does for next to nothing. The publication houses that understand this and adapt to it most effectively will have an immense competitive edge.

Feedback

The point-to-point capability of e-mail communication makes it possible for comment about a piece of scholarship to be delivered rapidly to the authors. Publications such as *The British Medical Journal* have incorporated this feature so that we can read the "article" and submit feedback immediately. It is then incorporated into the discussion of the article enriching (for the most part) the value of the work.

Updating

The obverse of feedback is the incorporation of the new ideas or criticisms into the work. We currently present information as if it were the last word and that one can draw a line under it and never return. Because updating of an Internet document is so easy, the incorporation of feedback should continue after posting. If, in the opinion of the authors, the comment is valid or needs to be answered, the change can be made and the updated version reposted. This is quite a departure from tradition and requires the rethinking of concepts such as dating the publication, acknowledgments, and even authorship. However, if we focus on what is desirable in the quest to provide the orthopaedic world with the best available information, these changes should be accommodated and welcomed. In reality individual research projects should be part of a "thread" with related projects leading into each other. Instead of the *Journal of Arthroscopy*, one might expect the same editorial guidance being used to manage a series of related threads posted on an "Arthroscopy Site."

The Uniqueness of the Internet

There must have been thousands of monks engaged in copying manuscripts when Gutenberg invented printing. One can easily imagine their reacting to the new invention with scorn over quality and an unshakable belief that real scholarship was handwritten. There is no fundamental difference between what can be printed and what can be hand copied. Yet the impact of printing was and remains enormous. Knowledge and scholarship changed from being the province of a tiny handful, and the energies released by that change transformed the world. The attributes of the Internet which we have outlined, based on the realities of computer operations, will, for identical reasons, change everything. The core knowledge of orthopaedic surgery is no longer inaccessible to anyone except orthopaedists and residents in training, Anyone with enough motivation can access *Wheeless' Textbook of Orthopaedics* (**http://www.medmedia.com**) and learn as much about a specific subject as his doctor. That aspect alone could change the world of medicine, and there are innumerable other examples. Like the monks, we can argue semantics and wonder whether this is really different from that. Meanwhile a tidal wave of change is beginning. The Internet has enormous potential for helping us with our information needs, and it is up to the whole profession to make sure that potential is realized.

The problem, then, that all of us try to solve with our various IT systems, paper and electronic, is keeping up with the literature and obtaining just-in-time updates on specific subjects when we need them. The situation is complex and information alone is seldom enough to change our practice. Synthesis of many sources of information may be necessary to form a conclusion. The Internet-based electronic IT systems make it much easier to search out and obtain the best available scientific information. In this volume we show you how much has already been accomplished in this area and point up tasks that have yet to be undertaken. Our purpose is to assist you in obtaining the most personally satisfying answers to the problem of accessing and evaluating the information and discovering the consensus you need as an orthopaedic surgeon to make the best choices. And, perhaps, to underline the fact that not using information to the best of your ability is also a choice, an ethically indefensible one.

Using the Internet

One of the most daunting aspects of the Internet and of the computer world in general is the strange new names for strange new concepts. New meanings crop up for words we think we recognize, such as Web and browser. Worse is the alphabet soup of abbreviations which the cognoscenti like to scatter around as if everyone, of course, should know for what FTP, TCP/IP, and HTML stand. We are probably guilty of this ourselves, although the plan was to introduce every abbreviation with its full version and to make sure that every abbreviation is in the glossary. Added to this insecurity is the dread that somehow you can break the Internet or your computer! Some of us even pride ourselves in the inevitability of computer breakdown any time we try to use the infernal machine. We are therefore offering a digression into how the contents of the Internet are translated by your machine into something that you see on the screen as a Web page or Internet document. You don't need to read this if you are comfortable with how the computer and the Internet communicate. If it is the last thing you need to know, skip ahead to the section on Web sites. But we keep it short and it may help if you have a burning need to understand or a deep anxiety that you can somehow damage things.

Files

Everything the computer stores—text, music, pictures, or videos—is in the form of binary numbers arranged in files. Because a binary number is either on or off (1 or 0 for clarity), the computer has no shades of meaning for that piece of information. This is what contributes to the accuracy of computers: the fundamental information cannot be confused; it's either on or off. If you string binary numbers together, you can get larger numbers (see Table 1.3). For example, the binary number 1001 translates as 1 one, no twos, no fours, and 1 eight—total 9. A string of eight binary numbers can therefore represent any number from 0 to 255. 256 numbers is large enough to encode all the letters of the (Western) alphabet, all commonly used keyboard actions, and most symbols. So text is stored as a whole lot of binary numbers varying in value between 0 and 255 (decimal). If you want to decode what is actually stored in the computer, you have to know the American Standard Code for Information Interchange (ASCII) coding convention under which for some strange reason #65 stands for "A" and #97 for "a". If you want to see the full set of ASCII codes, see **http://www.asciitable.com/**. Fortunately, unless you are a geek

TABLE 1.3. Binary and decimal numbers.

Binary	1	0	0	1
Base 10	8s	4s 9	2s	1s

you never need to use this. Any computer program worth the name translates the ASCII code into text for you. The takehome point is that because the computer stores the information in on/off form, copying and presentation of information is very accurate.

So where does this information get stored? What is a "file" and how does the computer know where it begins and ends? Data storage media do vary from computer to computer, but for most of us the data are stored on the hard drive as little magnetic dots. Related information is stored as a file which basically is a long string of binary numbers in order. A computer maintains a directory that remembers where all the files begin and end and what they are called. Naming is important because you and the computer need to identify the file to use it and the computer needs to know what type of file it is. Since the files are really all the same (a long string of numbers) the computer needs to know how to interpret those numbers and translate them back into something we poor humans can actually value. If you have been involved in naming files in the WINDOWS™ operating system, you know that there is a name and a suffix. The name (sometimes) tells you what is in the file and the suffix tells you and the computer what type of file it is.

So when terms like "file server," "file transfer," or "open file" are bandied about, you should understand what is happening. When you want some information from the Internet, your computer sends a request for a certain file (long string of numbers). The request is passed over the Net to the computer that holds the file permanently in memory. This computer then "serves" the file by sending the exact string of numbers onto the Net. The file is broken up into packets and transferred over the Net until it reaches your computer where it is reassembled again into a file. This file, an exact copy of the string of numbers that was stored somewhere out there on the Net, is now opened by the program on your computer and the information contained in the file is displayed on your screen. If you have a slow connection, you may see some parts of an image arrive and be displayed by your browser before other parts. This is because the files arrive in packets. It's wonderful that it happens and it's wonderful that you don't have to understand it or worry about it. Certainly you don't have to worry about doing damage, because what gets to you is a copy of the file; the unchanged original is resident on some uncaring hard drive half-way across the world!

The simplest form of file that you are likely to encounter is the text file, which traditionally has the suffix .txt. These are essentially strings of ASCII code numbers that are translated directly into text. The word "and" in a text file would be coded 01100001, 01101110, 01100100 (in binary,

97,110,100 in decimal) but when the file was read by the appropriate program these three numbers would appear as "and"—without color, without formatting—in the default font of the computer. This seems rather dull and it may come as a shock that the vast majority of files on the Internet are text files. However, the text incorporates special instructions to specify formatting and display of the text. The instructions are in the form of tags or marks and the files are in Hypertext Markup Language or HTML.

HTML Files

We know that files are strings of numbers, but since we only can read them when they are converted into text let us consider only the text translation. So how do we get from a dull text file to a cool Web page if the files are fundamentally the same?

Embedded in the text are instructions to the program that is going to interpret the file. The easiest way to understand this is to start with a simple text file and build it into a Web page using HTML. We start with a text file containing the simple phrase: "OWL Orthopaedic Web Links Gateway to the Orthopaedic Internet." This is exactly what the text file would contain and all it would contain.

The basic idea of HTML is quite easy. Dotted around in the text are opening and closing "tags" that are denoted by being enclosed in ⟨ ⟩. The opening tag is in the form ⟨html⟩ and the closing tag is in the form ⟨/html⟩. Everything between these two tags is then affected in some way.

An HTML file always opens with the ⟨html⟩ tag to indicate that the file is an HTML file. It usually has two distinct parts, the head and the body. The head contains the title of the page and instructions that relate to the whole page such as the background color. The body contains the information that the file is intended to convey.

If we apply this to our text file, it will look like this:

⟨html⟩
⟨head⟩
⟨/head⟩
⟨body⟩
OWL Orthopaedic Web Links Gateway to the Orthopaedic Internet
⟨/body⟩
⟨/html⟩

Note that each tag is opened and closed. Therefore any instructions enclosed in the ⟨body⟩ ⟨/body⟩ tags will not apply to the head section and vice versa. In fact there is nothing in the head section. We should add a title. Now the head section will be

⟨head⟩
⟨title⟩What is OWL?⟨/title⟩
⟨/head⟩

If you copied this exactly to a text file editor on your computer, saved the file with the name "orthogate.htm," and then opened that file in your Internet browser, you would see this as a page, true a very dull page, but honestly that is all that is strictly necessary to convert a text file into a Web page!

We can't do anything about the content but we can jazz up the presentation. We can edit the text file until it looks like this:

⟨html⟩
⟨head⟩
⟨title⟩What is OWL?⟨/title⟩
⟨/head⟩
⟨body⟩
⟨h1 align="center"⟩⟨font face="Arial"⟩OWL ⟨br⟩
Orthopaedic Web Links⟨/font⟩⟨/h1⟩
⟨p align="center"⟩⟨font face="Arial"⟩Gateway to the Orthopaedic Internet⟨/font⟩⟨/p⟩
⟨/body⟩
⟨/html⟩

The additional tags are:

- ⟨h1 align = "center"⟩ Meaning that the text following will be aligned in the center of the page and will be in Heading 1 format (i.e., large and bold). The instruction is terminated by ⟨/h1⟩.
- ⟨font face = "Arial"⟩ Meaning that the next piece of text should be displayed using the Arial font. This is closed by the ⟨/font⟩ tag.
- ⟨br⟩ Denoting a line break. It is one of the few tags that doesn't need to have a close.
- ⟨p align = "center"⟩ Meaning begin a new paragraph. The new paragraph is aligned with the center of the page. The end of the paragraph is denoted by ⟨/p⟩.

No Web page is complete without a link to another Web page—how else could you surf? In this instance it would be reasonable to provide a link to the OWL site (**http://owl.orthogate.com**). You can do this by adding another tag to the file.

- ⟨a href="http://owl.orthogate.com"⟩OWL⟨/a⟩, the ⟨a⟩ ⟨/a⟩ tags enclosing the instructions stating that the text "OWL" is to be a link to the address owl.orthogate.com. The "href" tag indicates that the next piece of text is an address and the part enclosed in quotes is that address.

How about an illustration? You might think it would be impossible to put a graphic file into a text file and you would be correct. What you put in are text instructions about inserting an image file.

• ⟨img src="owlogo.jpg"⟩ ⟨img denotes that an image will be placed here. The src="owlogo.jpg" indicates that the source of the image is the file owlogo.jpg The .jpg suffix indicates that this is an image file in JPEG format. The address indicates that the image file is in the same folder as the HTML file.

The completed file now looks like this:

⟨html⟩
⟨head⟩
⟨title⟩What is OWL?⟨/title⟩
⟨/head⟩
⟨body⟩
⟨h1 align="center"⟩⟨font face="Arial"⟩⟨a href="http://owl.orthogate.
   com"⟩OWL⟨/a⟩⟨br⟩
Orthopaedic Web Links⟨/font⟩⟨/h1⟩
⟨p align="center"⟩⟨img src="owlogo.jpg"⟩⟨/p⟩
⟨p align="center"⟩⟨font face="Arial"⟩Gateway to the Orthopaedic
   Internet⟨/font⟩⟨/p⟩
⟨/body⟩
⟨/html⟩

With all these tags the text file is beginning to look unreadable and unintelligible. However, we have seen that most of it is about display; the content is unchanged. If you are obsessional or fascinated by the nuts and bolts of Web pages, you can type that in on Notepad, save it as an .htm file, and open it in a browser. If you have a copy of the OWL logo in the same folder on your computer, then the page will look very much like this (see also Figure 1.2).

The reasons for this digression into geek-speak can be summarized as follows:

1. You must understand what a file is unless you are going to be purely passive and never create or store one.

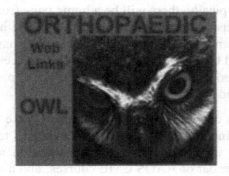

OWL
Orthopaedic Web Links

FIGURE 1.2. Output of a simple HTML file

2. The on/off nature of computer storage and transmission of information makes it superhumanly accurate.
3. You cannot damage the source files. Very often they are thousands of miles away and you deal with copies.
4. Text files are very simple, containing textual information with almost no formatting.
5. Hypertext Markup Language (HTML) files are text files with tags added to improve the format.
6. When you look closely there is nothing very mysterious about this stuff. The details are quite easy to understand; it looks scary *en masse*.

Best of all you don't have to deal at this level of detail even if you want to write Web pages. All of the particulars can be handled by Web page editing programs (see Chapter 5).

Web Sites

Web sites are collections of files maintained on a file server somewhere and registered with the powers that rule the Internet (**www.register.com**) as a domain. As mentioned earlier, a domain on the Internet is in reality a numerical address. Typically the files will be a collection of HTML files, graphics, sound, and video files all linked together and all serving some sort of common function. Nowadays many of the more sophisticated Web sites are database-driven so that the files that are sent to you are created on-the-fly in response to the requests that you send. A prime example of this would be the PubMed MEDLINE journal citations search site. What is sent to you depends on the search parameters you send to PubMed (**http://www.ncbi.nlm.nih.gov/PubMed/**).

Most Web sites are constructed as a hierarchy of interrelated pages connected by links. Typically, there will be a home page from which you can navigate to the parts of the site that interest you. The home page of the AAOS is an excellent example (Figure 1.3), showing navigation aids that can be used to send the user to dozens of different places in the Web site. They are subdivided into categories as can be seen from the tabs along the top, bottom, and side.

Medical Education contains online CME courses, case presentations, library resources including AAOS journals and links to other published material, online evaluation programs, information about the annual meeting, the calendar of AAOS CME courses, and a catalog of AAOS educational resources such as videotapes and CD-ROMs. Also in this section are tutorials on using the Internet.

Patient/Public Information has links to fact sheets, brochures, and booklets prepared for patient information by the AAOS. There is also a fa-

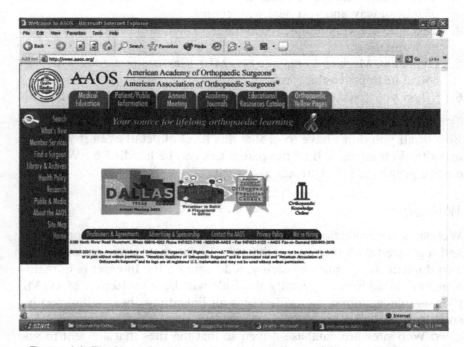

FIGURE 1.3. The Home Page of the American Academy of Orthopaedic Surgeons

cility for finding a surgeon (AAOS member) in various communities and geographical locations throughout the world.

The Annual Meeting portion of the site has full information about upcoming and past meetings including registration and travel information and the abstracts of presentations.

Academy Journals has links to *The Journal of the AAOS* and to JBJS.

Educational Resources has links to material prepared for this purpose by the academy including books, CD-ROMs, videotapes, self-assessment exams, courses, and so on.

The *Orthopaedic Yellow Pages* section gives access to a number of orthopaedic supply corporations.

Other links from the side of the page give access to

- a search engine for the site,
- specific services for members of the academy including creating your own Web site,
- archives and library functions,
- a list of policy statements,
- information about AAOS research projects,
- public relations material,
- AAOS structure, and
- site map.

In all there are nearly one hundred parts of the Web site that can be reached directly with one click from the home page.

Another increasingly common access point to a Web site is the Splash Page. This is a page with almost no information in it except a link to the home page. There may be an elaborate animated graphic to attract and hold the attention. This page has two main functions: to be attractive to search engines and to foster the interest of users so they will visit the site. Pages that are attractive to search engines have some likely search strings on them in the title, in the keywords, and as text, but very little else. More details of the operations and features of the search engines are given in Chapter 4.

Your Browser

If you have used the Internet for almost anything except e-mail, you have very likely used a browser. It is not a herbivore; it is the program resident on your machine that interprets the HTML file which you have collected from the Internet and opened. There are many browser programs, all with very similar functionality. The two most popular programs are

Internet Explorer (from Microsoft) and Netscape. If you are using a browser supplied by your Internet service provider (e.g., AOL), it will do the same things, but you may need to refer to the help files to find out exactly how to do some of the functions detailed below. Both Netscape and Internet Explorer (IE) are available free of charge. Netscape browser options can be found at **http://browsers.netscape.com/browsers/main. tmpl**. IE comes with any version of the WINDOWS™ OS later than WINDOWS™95. The most recent version of IE can be downloaded from **http://www.microsoft.com/windows/ie/default.asp.**

Although you may have used a browser, you may not have understood exactly what it does. Fundamentally, the program takes the text that is contained in the HTML file and displays it according to the instructions provided by the tags which are also contained in the HTML file. If the HTML file contains the text ⟨font face="Times New Roman" size = "4"⟩ Orthopaedic Surgery⟨/font⟩, when the browser program gets to that part of the file it will display the words "Orthopaedic Surgery" using the font Times New Roman (size 4) which is Orthopaedic Surgery. This may not seem very different from the way a word processing program works, but the underlying concept of a browser program is that it achieves an astonishing level of complexity from the very simple file structure of a text file. Since a text file can be read by nearly all computers, no matter what their OS might be, the browser programs have been very liberating. We have kept our examples of HTML tags simple, but they can get very complicated indeed. These complex instructions are all interpreted by the browser programs, in a manner invisible to the user. However, it is worth knowing about some special features of browsers.

Configuring Your Browser

Although the browser is most often automatically configured when you set it up, this may not be satisfactory forever. If you are using the WINDOWS™ OS, it won't function without Internet Explorer. If you prefer using Netscape as the default browser, you may have to reconfigure. You also have to do this if you change your Internet service provider or if you want to change the home page that your browser opens to automatically when you start the program. Figure 1.4a shows a typical browser setup

In IE the configuration options are found under the Tools menu. Select Internet Options to see the configuration dialog boxes. IE offers options under many different headings. The General and Programs tabs are the ones most often used (shown in Figure 1.4b). In Netscape open the Edit Menu and select Preferences to change the configuration options, as shown in Figure 1.4c.

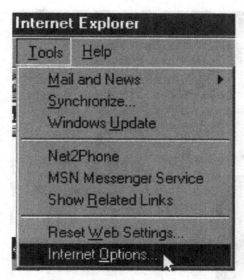

FIGURE 1.4a. Browser configuration. The Internet options in the tools menu of Internet Explorer

Updating

It used to be that updating a browser program was an exciting opportunity to use the Internet in new ways. The original browsers offered text and static graphics files only. With each update new heights of cool were scaled as streaming video, Java capabilities, and gif animation were added. Nowadays the sober truth is that updates are more and more necessary as virus designers seek to exploit weaknesses in the design of the browser and e-mail programs.

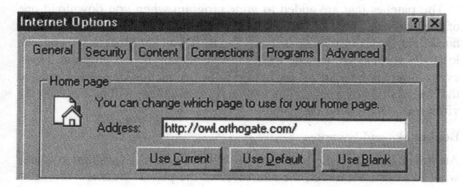

FIGURE 1.4b. The general tab in the Internet Options of Internet Explorer allows you to change the home page

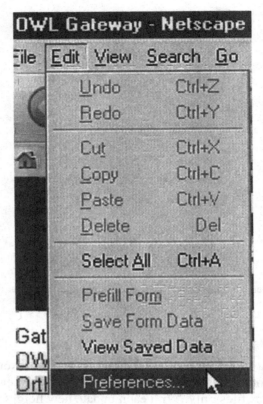

FIGURE 1.4c. The preferences tab in the edit menu of Netscape

Microsoft thinks it is so important that updating is one of the items on the IE tools menu (Figure 1.5). You can set it up so that you will be reminded about updates or e-mailed when a critical improvement is made.

The patches that are added to your program when you download one of these updates may be a source of concern and some software maintenance experts advise against using them. If you feel that way, you can look out for and acquire the most current version of the program. However, there will be a longer lag between the production of a new virus and the introduction of a new protected version than there will be between the virus introduction and the patch.

Bookmarks and Favorites

As you surf through the Internet you will come across sites that you may want to revisit. However, the addresses of the pages of interest are difficult to remember. Browsers offer the option of storing the addresses and

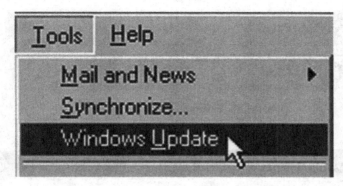

FIGURE 1.5. Internet Explorer, Windows updating

the titles of the pages. In Netscape these reminders are called "Book-marks" and in IE "Favorites." Because you might very soon have an un-wieldy collection of page addresses, both browsers offer ways to collect the addresses into folders.

In IE the Favorites function can be invoked from many parts of WINDOWS™ including the start menu in some versions. From Inter-net Explorer itself it can be opened by clicking on the Favorites icon in the toolbar. See Figure 1.6a. This results in the Favorites list being per-manently displayed in a panel to the left of the screen. To close the panel click on the X at the top right of the Favorites panel. The easiest way to view favorites is to click on the Favorites menu tab in IE. See Figure 1.6c. Whichever way you open the function, you will see a list of folders and selected sites. Often the manufacturer will start you off by providing folders with selected sites. To add the site the browser cur-rently has open simply click on "Add to Favorites." See Figure 1.6d.

Note in my list of favorites, shown in Figure 1.7, there is a folder called "OWL possibles." This is where I store addresses of sites that may be added to the OWL database of sites of orthopaedic interest. If I open the folder of OWL possibles (by clicking on it), a subset of "favorites" will

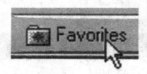

FIGURE 1.6a. Internet Explorer Favorites button

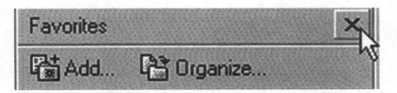

FIGURE 1.6b. Favorites panel closure button

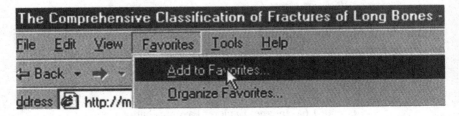

FIGURE 1.6c. The Favorites menu tab of Internet Explorer

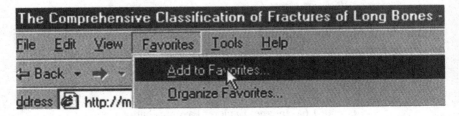

FIGURE 1.6d. Add to favorites

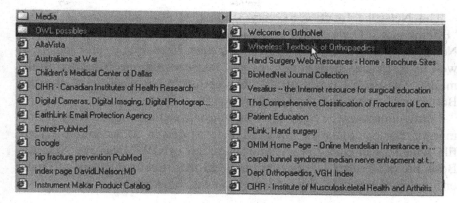

FIGURE 1.7. Subfolders in favorites

be displayed. To check out one of the sites (e.g., *Wheeless' Textbook of Orthopaedics,* Figure 1.8), I only need to position the cursor over the title (as shown in Figure1.7 right) and click for the page to load. What is displayed are the (understandable) titles, not the (forgettable) addresses.

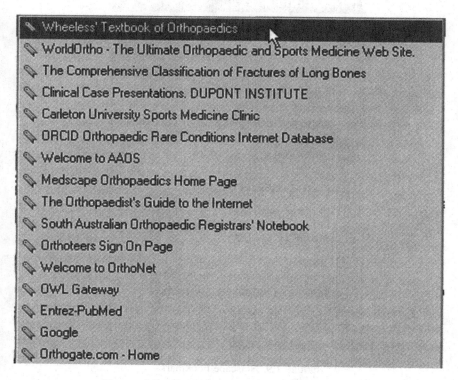

FIGURE 1.8. Wheeless' Textbook of Orthopaedics

The Netscape function is very similar. Useful addresses are called "Bookmarks." Once again some folders are provided—this time by Netscape—that contain links to various sites. If your computer runs IE as well as Netscape, the IE favorites will be imported into Netscape Bookmarks. The easiest way to start the function in Netscape is to open the Bookmarks menu, as shown in Figure 1.9.

For my purposes the Netscape Bookmark function is superior by a small margin. For one thing the bookmarks are stored in an accessible HTML file which I can edit. In fact the foundation of OWL was my Netscape Bookmarks file after I discovered in 1995 that it contained links to more orthopaedic sites than any other page I had come across.

Netscape Bookmarks Folders

To accumulate the sites I put together as the "Orthopaedic Surfboard," it was very easy to direct Netscape to each of those sites, bookmark the page, edit the bookmarks into a sensible order, then copy the corresponding segment of the bookmarks file.

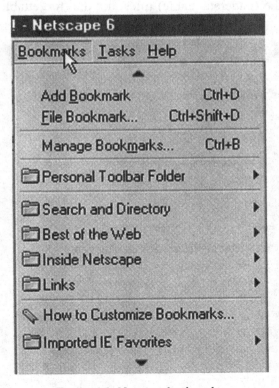

FIGURE 1.9. Netscape bookmarks

History

Both browsers have a history function that allows you to find the sites which you (or your kids) have been visiting.

In IE click the History icon on the toolbar (see Figure 1.10a).

A panel will open at the left of the screen similar to the screen shot. Note that my history is preserved back to two weeks ago. I open the folder for last Wednesday and see that I visited six sites that day. Each site is designated as a folder, and to see the actual pages I called up, you can open the folder. In this case the only page I opened on the OWL site that day was the home (Gateway) page (see Figure 1.10b). Note that the page is a link and the cursor is a hand. One click will take me to that page.

The History function in Netscape is opened by the keystroke Control H or by opening the Tasks Menu, then Tools, then History. It is similarly organized into folders corresponding to different days or time periods. Double click to open the selected page. See Figure 1.11.

Plug-Ins

Plug-ins are software programs that extend the capabilities of the browser in a specific way, giving you, for example, the ability to play audio samples or view video movies from within your browser. Plug-ins may be an integral part of the Web browser or you may have to download them separately. They include

- *Apple Quick Time* animation player,
- *Abobe Acrobat Reader,* which is needed to read PDF files,
- *Macromedia Flash Player* (animation),
- *Macromedia Shockwave Player* to display Web content that has been created by Macromedia Director Shockwave Studio, and
- *Real Player* for streaming audio, video, animations, and multimedia presentations.

FIGURE 1.10a. Internet Explorer History button

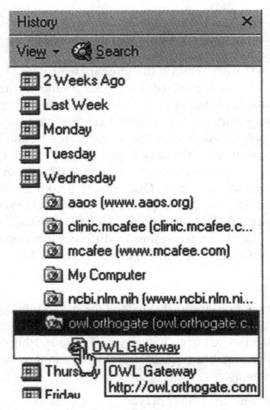

FIGURE 1.10b. Internet Explorer history

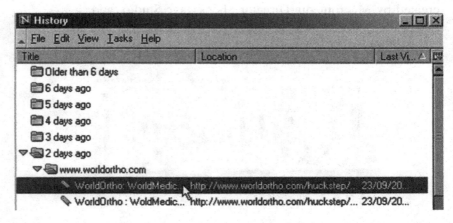

FIGURE 1.11. Netscape history function

Once a plug-in program has been loaded, your browser will respond to a call to use a media file in one of these formats by loading the plug-in and transferring control to it.

Cookies

Cookies are small files that can be inserted into your computer through the browser program when you visit a specific site (see Figure 1.12).When you revisit the site some information about your activities will be transferred back to the Web site computer. The best and least sinister example of this is the History function at PubMed. This will insert a cookie that keeps track of the searches you undertake. Then if you want to combine them, you can call up the History function and modify or combine previous searches. If you don't allow cookies to be placed on your computer, or if you have a firewall that will not allow them, you cannot use this function. At worst, cookies are used unscrupulously to record which pages you visited on a site. This information is then used to target you for specific advertising and presum-

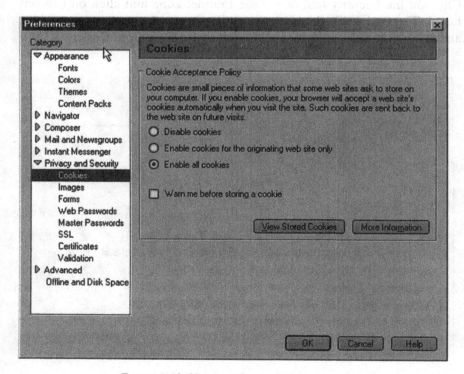

FIGURE 1.12. Netscape Cookies Dialog Box

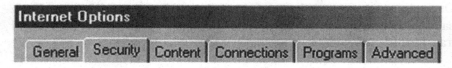

FIGURE 1.13a. Internet explorer options

ably could be used in even less desirable ways. If that possibility doesn't bother you and you are impervious to junk mail, then cookies may not be an issue. If not there are several levels of control that you can use.

In Netscape the options are found by opening Edit/Preferences, then Privacy and Security, and finally clicking on Cookies. As can be seen (Figure 1.12) the options include refusing all cookies, enabling some, or enabling all cookies. A useful function is, "Warn me before storing a cookie." If you are warned when visiting a site you don't trust, then you can refuse the cookie.

In IE Figure 1.13a open the Tools menu and select Internet Options. Click on the Security tab. Select the Internet zone and click on Custom Level (Figure 1.13b). Scroll down until you see the section on cookies and make your selections by clicking on the radio buttons (Figure 1.13c).

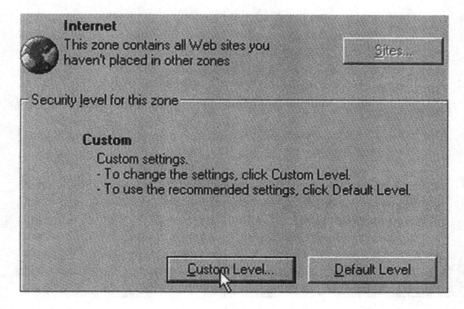

FIGURE 1.13b. Internet explorer options

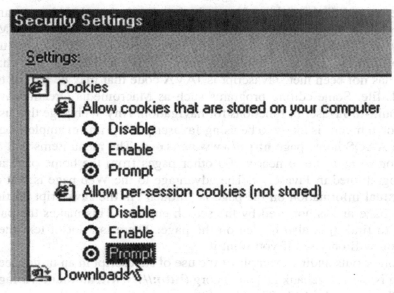

FIGURE 1.13c. Security selection, cookies

Internet Languages

JAVA and Javascript

This is another subject that you can skip unless the technical side of the Internet interests you. If you are concerned with putting up an elaborate page or want to know how some of the more dramatic effects are achieved, you may need to understand what JAVA and Javascript are. When a Web page loads with dropdown menus, cute animated displays, or a navigation bar that changes when the cursor hovers over it, the chances are that the page is using JAVA or Javascript. They are programming languages used to add display functions or interactions to a Web page. JAVA was developed by Sun Microsystems (**www.sun.com**) as a platform-independent language. It is closely related to C++ but has some important distinctions. The first is that JAVA programs (applets) will only run through a browser. The program instructions are loaded when the Web page is loaded, but from a different source. The JAVA code is interpreted by the browser to produce the desired effect. Since you have loaded the browser suited to your computer, the JAVA instructions will be interpreted correctly. So a standard set of instructions will produce the same effect on any machine. This is more clever than it sounds; most programs will only run on one type of machine.

The second distinguishing feature is that, by design, JAVA programs cannot load, edit, or delete anything in your computer's memory. Sun Microsystems challenged the hackers and virus designers of the cyber underworld to use JAVA to implant a virus or Trojan. Thus far this challenge has not been met. Javascript is JAVA code that may be part of the HTML file. Some editing programs such as Macromedia Dreamweaver have built-in Javascript functions for navigation. Any Web page that uses dropdown menus is likely to be using Javascript. A prime example would be the AAOS home page **http://www.aaos.org**. The menu items that allow you to navigate to nearly 100 other pages from the home page are all programmed in Javascript. The advantage to the Web page is that all the textual information on the page is "hidden" in the Javascript portion of the page and is not used by the search engines. This makes the page easier to find. It is also hidden on the page. There is a lot of text there that you will only see if you want it.

Another outstanding example of the use of Javascript in an orthopaedic setting is the Imagebank at Trauma.org (**http://www.trauma.org/imagebank/imagebank.html**). The classification tree that you follow down to identify the region and type of fracture of interest is a Javascript program.

Security

There is a great deal of free-floating anxiety about the security of information passed over the Internet. People who will hand over their credit card without a qualm or phone or fax their number are terrified that sending their card number over the Internet is an open invitation to the fraudulent. In reality it is quite difficult to intercept an e-mail message or the passage of this sort of information over the World Wide Web. The danger of someone steaming open envelopes or getting credit card numbers from the stubs in the trash can is greater. Another significant danger is that a hacker can get access to a store's database and find your credit card number that way. This may occur independently of how you sent in your credit card information in the first place.

However, since the messages do pass over the Internet through many different computers, there is a finite risk that they might be intercepted. To guard against this risk most sites that ask for sensitive information increase the security of the message by encrypting it. Any page whose address starts "https" invokes encryption both at your browser and at the server. Thus even if the message is intercepted it is unreadable unless the interceptor also has the encryption key.

Patients and the public expect that medical information is kept private.

It is also well accepted that physicians exchange information about patients in private letters (consults), in medical records, and in scientific communications. When you compare how easy it is for unauthorized individuals to look at a hospital or office chart as against how difficult it would be to intercept a specific message on the Internet, it may seem that privacy on the Internet is a nonissue. It isn't. Unless the local political system has issued clear guidelines you should take precautions before sending any confidential patient information over the Internet. This might include avoiding any identifying information. Encryption is even safer but requires the (secure) exchange of encryption keys ahead of time. If you are going to post anything about a patient on the Internet, the best thing to do would be to obtain their consent and provide them with the address of the site where their information will be available. In some jurisdictions the concept of privacy has extended to X-rays, with individuals claiming that unauthorized display of their X-rays is an invasion of privacy.

Another security concern relates to hackers. These are individuals who exploit vulnerabilities in your operating system to gain access to your computer files. If you have an "always-on" system with connection to the Internet, your machine may be accessible. Many of the current viruses (Trojans) install a "backdoor" in your system allowing a hacker access. The best answer to this is a firewall system which is either a physical router that will only let through approved messages or a software system on your computer that does the same thing. When we changed from a phone modem to a cable modem system without a firewall we were immediately infected with viruses, which then spread to all the computers in our local area network at home. If you are considering setting up a LAN at home to share computer hardware such as scanners and printers, we advise you to get it set up by a professional who is paying attention to the security issue. Set up the LAN first and make sure it is functioning, then set up the Internet connection with a router acting as a firewall.

2
Connecting to the Internet

Quick Start to the Internet

What is required to get started? You should purchase a fully loaded computer with a modem and Internet software installed. Purchasing a computer with AOL or MSN installed by the manufacturer can make the connection fast and painless. A free year of connection time is usually offered at the time of the purchase. When the computer arrives home, the monitor, keyboard, and mouse are attached to the computer. The phone line is plugged into the modem of the computer. If you have purchased the computer with the free year of MSN installed, you simply hit the "connect" button and you are on the Internet. If you did not have the computer Internet connection configured at the store, you need to install the software by clicking on the "connect to the Internet" icon. The wizard will guide you through the rest of the connection. A toll-free number (the only free part of this procedure) will allow you to set up an account with your credit card. Starting with MSN (Microsoft Network) or AOL (America Online) will allow the neophyte to immediately access the Internet with minimal fuss. AOL has a local phone number in most communities allowing you to dial up without long-distance phone charges. AOL has various plans that offer either a limited or unlimited number of hours of connection to the Internet. AOL, MSN, and others provide you with the most popular feature of the Internet, an e-mail address. The AOL software is also available free in the back of many computer trade magazines. On the downside of these ISPs, once you have subscribed, it is very difficult to cancel the subscription without cutting up your credit card!

Another alternative is to contact a local Internet service provider (ISP). Look in the phone book Yellow Pages under Internet service; it will usually list several companies that provide the connection service. It is usually best to get a recommendation from someone in your community who is happy using a local provider. The cable TV companies, as well as the phone companies, are getting into the business. Again, asking someone who is using the service in your area is recommended. The phone company provides fast, DSL (digital subscriber lines) Internet connection, but the service varies greatly depending on the distance from the booster node. The phone and cable companies, as well as the local service providers, have technical support personnel that will come to your home or office to configure the hardware and software to get you connected. This last option is the best solution for someone who is unfamiliar with the technical operation of a computer.

Practical Tip. Go to a computer or appliance shop, pick out a midrange desktop computer, buy the extended warranty and the MSN connection for a year (if it is available in your community), and you are ready to connect to the Internet. Investigate both the phone and cable companies that offer package deals with free installation. The best advice is to jump in, get your feet wet, and then after a trial period and some experience, you can decide to change your method of access to the Internet. However, remember that some providers have a nasty reputation of making it difficult to cancel your subscription.

Practical Tip Try not to waste time surfing the Internet. There are enough distractions when you are attempting to find some useful information; don't get waylaid by mindless surfing. They call it surfing for a reason. It's fun but superficial. On the other hand, it may be useful as a newcomer to the Internet to check out the Orthopaedic Surfboard at **http://condor.sechrest.com/clough/book/orthosurf.htm** to discover a taste of the vast amount of useful orthopaedic information that is available.

The Details

In the beginning (that's way back six or seven years ago in cyberspace time), connecting to the Internet was a daunting job. Now, with many computer magazines that you can pick up in the corner store, the ubiquitous AOL CD will be free in the back of the magazine. Either this CD or a recent computer purchase will have you up and running.

Hardware

The question of whether to purchase a Mac or a PC is still hotly debated, but usually only by the Macintosh users. The fact is that most business is done on a PC. If you need to do high-quality graphics or digital video editing, then consider a Mac; otherwise stick to what the rest of the world is using, a PC. All the brands have the same basic components. Go for the best service; Dell, Compaq, Toshiba, or Gateway. You get more bang for your buck with a desktop, but if you travel or do presentations you need a laptop as well. If you are going to do digital video capture from your arthroscopy camera, go with Sony products. The best advice for the power user is to buy the top of the line, since this will be the bottom of the line in about 18 months. After that, the $5,000 laptop will be good for word processing. If you are doing PowerPoint presentations and digital photography, get the fastest processor, that is, 800 MHz or 1 gig clock speed and max out the amount of RAM: 256 is minimum. A large hard drive, 30 gig, helps, but most of the information is going to be dumped off the laptop to the desktop after using it. If you are purchasing a laptop because you expect to travel with it, this may influence your choice of connection to the Internet. Early on, connection via a high-speed cable modem, ISDN, or DSL was only practicable at home or the office. However, some hotels now have an Ethernet connection in the room so it's not cut and dried.

Connecting the Desktop

When you purchase a new computer from any of the recognized computer stores, such as Best Buy, CompUSA, Future Shop, Gateway, or online at Dell **www.dell.com**, or Sony **www.sony.com**, the basic model (as low as $1,000) will have a modem and software installed to allow you to make a connection in about a half-hour. For the Internet only, a low-end (under $1,000) computer will suffice. If you plan on using the computer for presentations, the best advice is to buy the fastest available machine with the largest hard drive and at least 256 Mb of memory. If you are going to do digital editing, go for a minimum of 256 Mb memory and even 512 Mb to make the editing process less painful. The rationale for buying the fastest machine currently available is that the half-life of a laptop about two years.

The modem is the hardware that allows you to plug the phone line into the computer. Most computers come with a 56K modem that allows rapid transfer of e-mail messages, but is slow for multimedia. To get a high-speed connection at home, you need either a cable TV modem or DSL from the phone company. If you have a cable TV in your house, you need to contact the local cable company to get a high-speed modem (really just a router). This will give you high-speed access and an e-mail address. The other option for home use is the DSL, provided by your phone company. Again you have to contact the phone company to see if this is available in your area. It also helps to check with other customers in the area to see if they are pleased with the service. In most situations, you have to take what is available. I have both services and find the cable modem to be more consistent and reliable.

For your office you can have a high-speed Integrated Services Digital Network (ISDN) line installed by the phone company. This is expensive, but if there are multiple users in the group the cost can be spread around.

All new computers have software installed that will hook you up to America Online, Microsoft Network, or Prodigy in about 10 minutes. You simply click on the "Connect to the Internet" and the computer dials a toll-free number. Follow the instructions, give your credit card number, and you are connected. The browser (Internet Explorer and Netscape) will allow you to connect to the Internet sites by typing in the URL (uniform resource locator) of the site that you would like to visit. To avoid typing that long name again, go to "Favorites" on the dropdown menu and add the site to your favorites. Create a new folder for the groups of sites that you visit often, such as digital photography, orthopaedic university Web sites, and so on.

To set up the e-mail connection, follow the prompts on the screen. Select an e-mail address carefully; it may follow you around for many years. I have seven different addresses that I have accumulated over the years. I stopped one of my original addresses and still find it listed in orthopaedic organizations that I forgot to notify of the change. It seems to be easier to hang on to the old addresses rather than dropping them and not having people locate you.

How you connect to the Internet for the first time depends on a number of factors; cost, convenience, your location, what you want to use the Internet for, and how fast you want the connection to be.

Using the Internet

The primary value of the Internet is in providing information and communication. Here are some of the other things that you, as an orthopaedic surgeon, can use the Internet for, with comments on how this relates to the connection choice.

In Your Office

If patient information is the only use for the Internet in your office, you could get by with a dedicated phone line (and computer) in the waiting room. However, it would be an advantage to have "painless" connection for this use and this means fast. A cable or DSL connection to ensure that the information comes from the Internet very speedily will reduce anxiety on the patient's part. Most times you will want an Internet connection for your office too. The best solution is an office LAN connected to the Internet by a fast cable or DSL connection. Make sure that more than one station on the LAN can get access to the Internet at the same time. And also make sure you have a firewall if any of the computers on the LAN have confidential information. If you use the Internet during day-to-day activity in the office, either to look up information and the literature or to connect with the HIS (Hospital Information System) of your institution, you need a LAN and a fast-shared connection. A LAN will have the added advantage that files can be shared between workstations in the office and that each computer can be connected to such peripherals as printers and scanners through the LAN.

From the Hospital

Usually you have no control over this type of use. However, if you are asked to give advice from a clinician's point of view to the Hospital Information Systems (HIS) people, you should keep the following points in mind. Clinicians will need to access the Internet from anywhere in the hospital: wards, ER, OR lounge, library, or medical records. So access should be available from virtually every computer on the HIS system. Security should be thorough but user friendly. The Internet connection should be fast and through a firewall. Connection from the HIS to your office is also a prime consideration. If you have any choice, steer the hospital towards an intranet system for the main HIS; since this uses the Internet protocols for transfer of information, it makes access to the information you need from outside the system much easier.

Home Use

The Internet is entertaining as well as informative. It is also a great resource for finding information about travel, investing, and things to buy. It is an unparalleled educational resource, and children who do not have Internet access have an educational handicap. If your main use for Internet access is at home, then a simple telephone modem connection to a local ISP or to one of the multiple outlets (AOL or MSN) will be fine. In time, as more members of the household use the Internet, there will be conflicts over access and who uses the computer. You may therefore expect eventually to move up to a home network (LAN) and a fast connection that can be shared between users. This will be cable or DSL. Resist pressure to get a fast connection simply so that music files can be downloaded quickly! These files have a high incidence of virus infection that will then spread around your home network.

Traveling

If you plan to carry your laptop computer with you and to access the Internet from many different places, then you need an Internet connection with multiple outlets. Some local ISPs are part of a worldwide network that will allow you access from different points (iPass). However, some local ISPs will not allow you to send on messages that come from another server on the Internet. Thus if you are in Ottawa and your normal server is in Kamloops, a sent e-mail message must travel back to Kamloops over the Internet before it can be forwarded. The originators of nuisance messages (Spam) often conceal the origin of these messages by forwarding. As a result ISPs may block any forwarded messages including your legitimate ones. What this means is that when you are traveling you can receive e-mail through iPass but not send it. By contrast, if you connect via AOL, Earthlink, Mindspring, or MSN you get a local access number for many places throughout the country and even the world. Once signed on through that you can send and receive e-mail. AOL has access numbers in nearly all countries, but MSN and Earthlink are not so universal. IPass (**www.ipass.com**) has 11,000 local connections around the world, similar to AOL. These two services are the only ones that provide such widespread local phone connections for the traveler. You should check with your local ISP to see if it provides coverage with iPass and allows you to send messages this way.

E-Mail

If all you want is e-mail access to the Internet, you can obtain a free e-mail address by signing on to Hotmail (in the Microsoft organization), Yahoo, or many other providers. If you can get connected to the Internet by some other means (e.g., at an Internet café), then you can send and receive mail by connecting to the Hotmail site **www.hotmail.com** and supplying your user name and password. This is a good solution for travelers who want to be able to stay in e-mail contact, but it does mean you have to use someone else's Internet connection, so it isn't a solution for Internet connection at home.

Cost

There is a bewildering variety of ways to pay for Internet connection. Once connected, the charges may continue based on time connected or in some circumstances, the amount of information transmitted. This is obviously a prime concern and new users (newbies) will need to discuss rates with those who offer to provide Internet service. Most ISPs will provide a variety of rates from ones that limit connection to a few hours per month to more expensive ones that provide unlimited connection time. Unless you plan to surf the Internet for entertainment you may well want to start with a cheap connection and find out how much time you spend connected. There are ways to limit your time online. For example, after you have received all your e-mail messages you can close the connection, read the messages and write your replies, then go back online to send them. This takes much less connection time than staying online for the whole time.

Support

Sooner or later the Internet will make you tear out your hair. It is so enormously complex, it is amazing it works at all. When you want answers to questions about viruses, service interruptions, slow connection, or missing messages, the quality of support provided is important. In general the bigger the ISP organization the better, but the more remote the support site is. You can't just drag your computer into AOL, slam your fist on the counter, and say, "You fix the %@#$ thing." However, most ISPs do have phone support where you can speak to an expert and be guided through the remedy. It helps to have two phone lines for this exercise as you can test the solution before ending the phone call. If you want the personal touch, then a local ISP may be best for you.

Summary

Accessing the Internet, especially for the first time, is daunting. To summarize the options:

- local Internet service provider is an organization with a local office that will connect your computer to its local Internet server through a phone modem;
- cable/DSL/ISDN connection is provided by the phone company or the TV cable service provider. The connection is faster than by phone modem. The financial arrangements can be more complicated with bundles including phone service or cable TV service;

TABLE 2.1. Different methods of connection to the Internet.

	Local ISP	Cable/DSL	Multiple outlet	Hotmail
Cost	Varies. Usually fewer options	Varies. May affect phone and TV service costs	Varies according to time spent connected	Free
Features	Full service	Full service	Full service	E-mail only
Support	Local	Remote	Remote	Web based
Portability	Often none	None	Good	Excellent

- multiple outlets are available through providers AOL and MSN who supply Internet access just like local ISPs but have outlets in many different locations. This is a great advantage if you travel a lot and need to use the Internet en route; and
- Hotmail is a free e-mail service that is provided if you have Internet access by other means.

Table 2.1 summarizes the choices and implications.

Servers and Back Up

Back up, back up, and back up. It is not if, but when and how bad your computer crash or virus injection is going to be. Back up your information regularly. There are many different ways to back up. The most efficient way is to establish a cable connection between your laptop and desktop. Keep the important files, such as the PowerPoint slides and your clinical images, backed up on both computers. Backing up the data on Zip discs, CDs, or tape should further protect the desktop. After you start to accumulate a collection of Zips or CDs you will need to investigate other backup options. The best and most secure method is to use a RAID server to connect both the laptop and desktop. The server has multiple connected hard drives, a huge storage capacity, and can be further protected by tape backup. If one hard drive on a RAID server goes down, it is removed, replaced, and no data are lost. Compare that to the loss of one of your hard drives on the desktop, where all the data on that drive are lost. Each time you complete a project on either the laptop or desktop the data are transferred to the server. The next time that you need the image, it can be searched for on the server and transferred to the laptop. This server can also be used for a wireless network, so that you can move about the house with the laptop still connected to the server. This allows you to access the server files and the high-speed Internet connection

The medium of backup, however, is less important than the protocol you use to actually do it. In addition to the hardware you choose you need to consider the following:

- Choice of which folders you are going to back up. You can simplify this by keeping everything that you create in one folder (e.g., My Documents in WINDOWS™ 95+). Then when it comes time to backup you only need to remember one folder.
- Schedule of how often you do this.
- Software to select the files and folders you are backing up. Some software can set up an automatic schedule or prompt you to do it. For a review of backup software see
  - CNET Backup review (**http://www.cnet.com/software/0-806180-7-2376963.html**);
  - Backup Freeware (**http://www.freestuffer.com/software/backup.html**);
  - Backup Scheduler 98 (Cibeo) (**http://www.cibeo.com/software_store/backup_scheduler_98/default.htm**);
  - Hyper-Galaxy Software/shareware index (Backup) (**http://www.hyper-galaxy.com/Back-Up/**);
  - Backup Wolf (**http://www.lonewolf-software.com/backupwolf.htm**);
  - Column on Backup (**http://www.contracostatimes.com/computing/columnists/yael_liron/stories/o25yael_2001032 5.htm**).
- Storage for the backup material. If you feel the risk is attack on the system through viruses or hacking, then it doesn't matter where you store the backup discs. If, however, you factor in the risk of theft, fire, or flood, then you should store the backup material at a site geographically remote from the computer.

There are some ways to back up your material online. @Backup will encrypt your selected files and store them on a secure site. You can restore them to any computer if you have the password and encryption key (**http://www.backup.com/**).

Software

The ubiquitous operating system on the PC is Microsoft WINDOWS™. There are other options such as Linux, but for the nontechnical user they are not practical. The latest version, Windows XP, has by far the most stable platform. One word of advice: don't upgrade. Buy a new computer with the new OS installed. Also buy the computer with the Office 2000 suite already installed; it saves a lot of time and configuration. Office has all the programs that you need: Word, Excel, PowerPoint, Access, Internet Explorer, and Outlook. Word is the word-processing program, Excel the spreadsheet, PowerPoint the presentation tool, Access the database, Internet Explorer the browser for the Internet, and Outlook the personal information manager including e-mail.

The only other software that you need is image manipulation and archiving. PhotoDeluxe (**www.adobe.com**) or PhotoImpact (**www.ulead.com**) comes with most digital cameras or scanners. The other program that you need is one to archive images and do a slide show. PhotoImpact Explorer (**www.ulead.com**) allows you to view the thumbnails of images in a folder. It also will do basic imaging manipulation, such as crop, lighten/darken, and rotate. Image access is an excellent searchable database, but is no longer supported by **www.scansoft.com**. A good alternative to this program is the thumbsplus program (**www.thumbsplus.com**). This will display the thumbnails, assign keywords, and allow searching. Lightview (**www.lview.com**) is a program that edits and also archives images. The professional program for digital still imaging is Adobe PhotoShop (**www.adobe.com**). This is a very complex program, and for most amateurs is not worth the money.

Digital video editing can be done with Adobe Premier (**www.adobe. com**) or Ulead video editor (**www.ulead.com**). The concept that seems to work for me is to stick to Microsoft and Adobe products and there will be minimal conflicts. Software programs have a bad habit of interfering with each other, and you have to resist the urge to download some hot new application from the Internet that will crash your system. Use only one of the imaging programs at a time to avoid the conflicts.

The final word on software is to install and run one of the virus protection agents, either McAfee or Norton antivirus. See the section on viruses.

Practical Tip. Avoid downloading some new program from the Internet that often causes conflicts in your system. If you are prone to doing this, install a program called GoBack (**www.goback.com**). This allows you to revert your computer to the functional state before you messed it up with the new program. Windows XP now has this installed as a system restore function. This can be found under programs—accessories—system tools–restore system.

3
The Internet and the Orthopaedic Surgeon

Introduction

The orthopaedic surgeon uses the Internet to find information quickly, to communicate with other surgeons in his field, and to occasionally ask for help in managing a difficult or unusual case. After the dot.com and e-commerce shake up, the Internet is returning to its two primary functions, finding information fast and communicating with people. The tradition of the Internet has been that the information is free and available to everyone. When people discovered that you could not easily sell information, a different marketing model was developed. Advertising banners on the site supported the organization, archived issues were sold, and more detailed information required membership in the organization. Conventional suppliers of information, such as Encyclopedia Britannica (**http://www.britannica. com/**) and professional associations, such as the American Academy of Orthopaedic Surgeons (**www.aaos.org**) both supply free high-quality information and charge for special services. The traditional book publishers are still searching for the best model to provide online content. It is clear that the Internet and computer are not going to completely replace paper to access information. Books will still flourish, as many people still like to turn paper pages and read their information from a book.

But what can the Internet offer the orthopedic surgeon?

E-Mail

E-mail is what usually prods the traditional orthopaedic surgeon to get started using the computer and the Internet. Nothing is more embarrassing than being asked for your e-mail address and having to admit you don't know or even have one. Services such as AOL make this introduction to e-mail and the Internet fast and easy. This allows one to send and receive brief, and not so brief, messages to one's friends, family, and colleagues. Most e-mail programs make it simple to send, receive, and reply to messages. With e-mail the surgeon can exchange clinical information, including X-rays, to obtain consultations and opinions. Professional associations use e-mail to notify the surgeon of activities of the association. Hospitals can notify staff members of meetings and activities.

The difficulty is in organizing the messages for retrieval and action. Personal organizing programs such as Outlook combine the scheduling and addresses, to do tasks and e-mail all in one program.

The greatest drawback for older surgeons is the keyboard; most are simply not comfortable with typing, and consequently messages tend to be two-finger brief missives. One solution is to dictate the responses, and have your secretary type and send an e-mail message on your behalf.

MEDLINE Searches

Information retrieval is the most revolutionary aspect of the Internet. The process of a MEDLINE search used to be controlled by the medical librarian at the university or in the hospital. Now, instead of a visit to the library, you can be three clicks away from conducting your own search at home at 11 PM at night. The fastest way to access MEDLINE is directly through PubMed at **http://www4.ncbi.nlm.nih.gov/PubMed/**. These long names do not have to be typed in, but can be found in your bookmark list that is saved when you visit a site. (See Chapter 1.) Searching MEDLINE is a skill that must be learned and practiced. (See Chapter 4.) Only too often a search will produce an enormous list of citations, which may not even include the ones that are most relevant to your subject. We revisit this subject later in Chapter 4.

Most of latest journal articles may be read online. The *Journal of Arthroscopy* (**www.arthroscopyjournal.org**) posts the full text article with images and is free to all subscribers. The *Journal* site may also be searched for articles from the past several years. Each month the *Journal of Arthroscopy* e-mails subscribers a list of the table of contents of the latest *Journal*. The articles are hyperlinked to the Web site so that with a click of the mouse the full text article appears. Never has it been so easy to keep up to date. This is one of the benefits of a subscription to the *Journal of Arthroscopy* and is a membership benefit of the Arthroscopy Association of North America (**www.aana.org**) or the International Society of Arthroscopy, Knee Surgery, and Orthopedic Sports Medicine (**www.isakos.com**).

Remote File Access

If you have permission and the right password, files on other computers may be accessed by FTP (file transfer protocol). The software for these programs is inexpensive, and can be downloaded to your computer. An example of this type of program is Cuteftp available at **www.cuteftp.com**. This program allows you to connect to another computer using your ISP. WS-FTP has a limited edition version that is available free to educational and nonbusiness home users. There is also a full version, which can be evaluated for free for 30 days. Either can be downloaded from **http://www.ftpplanet.com/download.htm**. Figure 3.1 shows a sample FTP page.

When the FTP program is opened the remote computer is on the right side and the local on the left side of the screen. The file that is on the local computer is copied to the remote computer and the transfer takes place. The speed of the transfer depends on your type of connection. With the DSL and cable modem connection the transfer is very quick. FTP allows you to transfer the larger files that you can't send by e-mail. You must have a password and access privileges to connect to the remote site.

Another popular way to access your office or hospital files is to use Windows commercial software such as pc anywhere, available from **http://www.symantec.com/pcanywhere**. This allows you to connect your computer at home with the office computer over a phone line. Some institutional firewall programs will block the use of this type of transfer. Using this software splits your computer screen into two, the remote computer on one side and your own computer on the other. The folders are opened up and the files transferred by copying the file from one computer folder to the other.

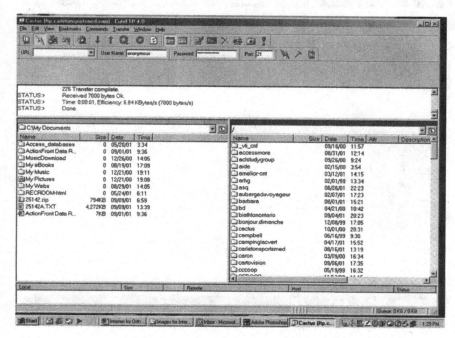

FIGURE 3.1. An example of a file transfer program (FTP)

Professional Association Information

Most professional organizations, such as the Arthroscopy Association of North America (**www.aana.org**), have a Web site to provide information about the association's activities, such as details of upcoming meetings, online registration for the meeting, and abstract submission. An example of a home page is shown in Figure 3.2. The button at the top, "web cast of the fall course 2000," leads to extensive coverage of the meeting with PowerPoint presentations and streaming video of surgical techniques.

The International Association of Arthroscopy, Knee Surgery and Orthopeadic Sports Medicine ISAKOS at **www.isakos.com** has information about the upcoming meeting, online abstract submission, paper and poster abstracts from the previous meeting, as well as an extensive listing of all the worldwide meetings related to knee surgery and arthroscopy. See Figure 3.3.

The American Academy of Orthopaedic Surgeons at **www.aaos.org** (home page shown in Figure 3.4), also has a detailed listing of the past and upcoming meetings. It is easy to register for the meetings, select the instructional courses, and arrange your housing. The newest addition to

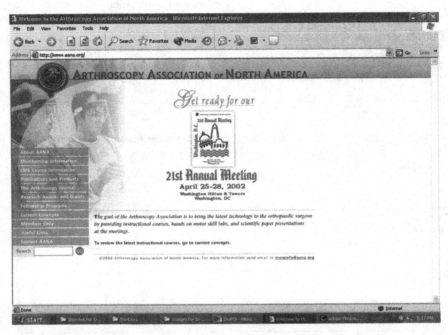

FIGURE 3.2. The home page of the Arthroscopy Association of North America

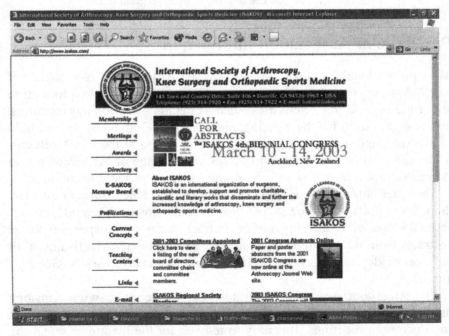

FIGURE 3.3. The home page of the International Society of Arthroscopy, Knee Surgery and Orthopaedic Sports Medicine

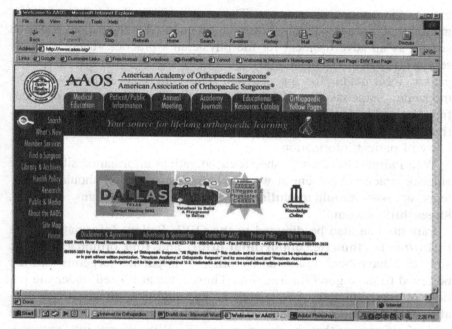

FIGURE 3.4. The home page of the American Academy of Orthopaedic Surgeons

the site is "Orthopaedic Knowledge Online." This is an extensive online multimedia program of current surgical practice.

The associations are also encouraging online abstract submission for annual meetings. This makes meeting management much easier. The program committee can review the abstracts online, grade them, and never have to wade through the stack of paper submissions.

OWL, Orthopaedic Web Links, the largest index of orthopaedic addresses on the Internet, has a list of orthopaedic organizations that maintain a Web site (**http://owl.orthogate.com/org.html**) and a short list of those that publish a major journal is included in this book (see Appendix 1, Journals).

Patient Information

Patient information seems to be the one area that is very actively used by the general public. In part because of our default, most of the information that orthopaedic patients read is not supplied by orthopaedic surgeons. In a survey of patients in a large orthopaedic practice in the USA, 80% had gone to the Internet for information prior to, or following, the visit to the orthopaedic surgeon. The main issue is the quality of information that is accessed. Some information directed at the patient is posted simply as an advertisement for the physician's practice. There are now services that will establish a physician Web site and link him to quality patient information for his patients. The American Academy of Orthopaedic Surgeons (**http://orthodoc.aaos.org/members.cfm**) provides free Web sites for its members. Active life networks (**http://www.activelifenetwork.com**) will set up and maintain a Web site with a rich library of patient information.

Web Partners have established focused patient information sites on the anterior cruciate ligament at **www.aclsolutions.com**, on shoulder problems at **www.shouldersolutions.com**, and knee problems at **www.kneesolutions.com**.

Patients can also be directed to the OWL Patient Information page (**http://owl.orthogate.com/orthpat.html**) and find orthopaedic Web sites that have been reviewed by other orthopaedic surgeons and are believed to have good information. These sites are listed under the patient information area of Appendix 1. The quality of these sites is usually related to the zeal of the volunteers who maintain the site or to the amount of money that the organization is willing to put into management of the site.

The main problem is that patients who use the Internet for medical information do none of these things. They don't go to the AAOS site because they don't know it exists, they don't go to their orthopaedic surgeon's site because there isn't one, and it wouldn't occur to them to visit professional association sites. What they do is use search engines, and what they find by that route is biased toward the slick and commercial and away from disinterested, scientifically based information.

In a review of Orthopaedic IT at the AAOS meeting in 2001 it was noted that patient information on the Internet was a major source of concern for orthopaedic surgeons. The studies found that patients who looked for information using the search engines were likely to find a poor-quality selection. "Although they all concluded that orthopaedic surgeons need to guide their patients, they did not, in fact, provide such guidance or offer links to sites where orthopaedic patients can find information that has been vetted by an orthopaedic surgeon" (Orthopaedic Information Technology, JFM Clough), Furthermore, amid the concern that the information a patient might find on the Internet would be incomplete, there was no sign of a study comparing that to the information a patient normally receives from his or her surgeon.

In a poster presentation to the Canadian Orthopaedic Association (Quality Assessment of Patient Information on Hip Arthroplasty, JFM

TABLE 3.1. Topics that should be covered in
orthopaedic patient information pages.

Condition	Nonoperative interventions	Operative interventions
Name	Investigations	Operative treatment
Synonyms	Nonoperative treatment	Indications for surgery
Pathological process	Risks of nonoperative	Risks of operative
Symptoms	treatment	treatment
Stages	Recovery time for non-	Surgical complications
Complications of the	operative treatment	Post-op rehabilitation
condition	Prognosis and outcomes	Post-op recovery time
Untreated prognosis	for nonoperative treatment	Post-op prognosis
	Complications of non-	Costs
	operative treatment	Location of surgical
	Costs	treatment center

Clough, 2000. Poster number 42. The Canadian Orthopaedic Association
55th Annual Meeting, June 2000), the subjects that should be covered in
a patient information document were identified. These are shown in Table
3.1 It was noted that none of 15 hip replacement patient information sites
surveyed in 2000 covered all these topics. Although the list may be incomplete it could be a starting point for reviewing and improving the information available to orthopaedic patients.

Physician Education and Online CME

A truly enormous amount of orthopaedic material has been posted on the
Internet even apart from the journal articles. Elsewhere in this book we
estimate that the Orthopaedic Internet is larger than 100,000 pages. It is
possible to find interesting and informative material on out-of-the-way
subjects. The frustration often is not knowing where it is or how to conduct a search. From core concepts like the American College of Rheumatology Guidelines for Management of Hip Osteoarthritis (**http://www.
rheumatology.org/research/guidelines/guidelines/oa-hip/oa-hip.html**)
to case presentations on rarities such as Gorham's Vanishing Bone Disease (**http://www.mcmaster.ca/inabis98/surgeryortho/clough0143/**), the
Internet has them all. For orthopaedic surgeons in isolated situations far
from a medical library, judicious use of the Internet for orthopaedic information is a tremendous step forward.

Online CME is one aspect that has not yet caught on with orthopaedic surgeons. Maybe it is because most surgeons are too busy and worn out to get their CME online at night and weekends. It may also be that many do not have high-speed Internet connections to take advantage of the multimedia content. The preferred method of updating their knowledge is to go to hands-on courses and annual meetings. Only 20% of physicians access any online continuing medical education. Medscape has provided online CME since its onset in 1995. The Arthroscopy Association tried online education and has been disappointed with the response. The entire fall course consisting of PowerPoint presentations with audio and video as well as surgical demos has been online at **www.aana.org** under "Webcast of the Fall Course 2000," but few members have taken advantage of this service. The major drawback of online PowerPoint presentations is the slow speed of a traditional modem connection. These multimedia files can only be successfully viewed with a fast broadband Internet connection. However, even the CDs of the entire course have not been wildly successful. At present, I think we realize what we can do with technology on the Internet, but there are too few computer-savvy surgeons with high-speed access to take advantage of this service.

In the future, this may change because interactivity is a key feature of the Internet. It is thus well suited to providing CME and testing or selftesting understanding and grasp of the material. The medium deserves teaching efforts tailormade to take advantage of its special attributes, not just transfers from paper or presentations.

The online medical CME sites are listed at **http://www.netcantina. com/bernardsklar/cmelist.html.**

The American Academy of Orthopaedic Surgery is the only orthopaedic association with three courses:

Post-Operative ACL Rehabilitation Course,
Rotator Cuff Diagnosis and Treatment, and
Nonoperative Treatment of Knee Osteoarthritis.

The CME center for the Academy is at **http://www3.aaos.org/courses/ welcometoaud.cfm.**

The CME center at Medscape may be found at **http://cmecenter.medscape.com/Home/CMEcenter/CMEcenter.html.**

The Medscape site also lists the coverage of recent orthopaedic meetings at **http://www.medscape.com/Home/Topics/orthopaedics/orthopaedics. html.** Before you get to this page on Medscape you have to register, but it's free.

Johns Hopkins also has an online course on arthritis that offers CME credits for $20 (**http://www.hopkins-arthritis.org/course/oa51101/course.html**).

Orthopedics® online CME site has a number of courses on offer at **http://www.orthobluejournal.com/CMEarticles.asp.** CME credit is also offered by the Physician and Sportsmedicine site in collaboration with the American College of Sports Medicine (**http://www.physsportsmed.com/cme.htm**). Many other teaching sites are listed on the OWL teaching page (**http://owl.orthogate.com/Teaching_Sites/index.html**) but most of them do not offer CME credit.

University Orthopaedic Sites

Most orthopaedic teaching institutions have posted a Web page and these are valuable introductions to the work and personnel of the department. But posting the site needs to benefit the program in some direct way. Attracting high-quality applicants to the resident training scheme or to fellowships would be one obvious tangible benefit. Equally valuable would be contact from colleagues or referring doctors who may refer patients to a member of the staff or to the institution via the Web site. The Web site should also be used as a means of communication within the institution and showcase its research and teaching. Improving the quality of the Orthopaedic Internet by posting good orthopaedic content may add to the reputation of the program and uphold the institution's reputation for innovation and excellence. A dynamic Web site that truly reflects our vital and forward-looking specialty may be an advantage. Thus these sites should include an account of the curriculum and the fellowships available; contact information for faculty, residents and fellows; an account of research opportunities at the institution; a calendar of events and as much orthopaedic content as possible. A 2001 review of Canadian orthopaedic departmental Web sites showed that only a few met these criteria (**http://www.coa-aco.org/library/Clough_Articles/sept-lead.htm**).

Professional and Personal Web Sites

Establishing your presence on the Web will become more important in the future. Patients may log on to your site prior to their visit to the office. They will enter the necessary demographics for the staff, make an appointment that is at a suitable time for them, fill in the history portion of the chart (such as the subjective IKDC form), and read information that pertains to their complaint. The time in the office is now optimized, the forms are filled in, the history taken, and the patient is ready to interact with the physician. After the office visit when the treatment plan is outlined, the patient may revisit the office Web site to review the surgical options, the procedure, and the recommended rehabilitation for the operation. The process of developing a Web site tailored to your practice is now very easy using the AAOS Web site (**www.aaos.org**), the site developed by active life (**www.activenetwork.com**), or one that is built for you by a local Internet service provider. Both authors have availed themselves of the service provided by the AAOS and have Web sites at **http://orthodoc.aaos.org/DonJohnsonMD/** and **http://orthodoc.aaos.org/MylesClough/**.

Active life networks has started an interesting initiative of serial e-mails for your patients. The patient is e-mailed prior to surgery to review the pre-op instructions. Then a series of template e-mails is sent at regular weekly and monthly intervals to provide further information for the patient as he progresses through the rehab program. The follow-up outcome studies can be incorporated into this automated system.

Nonmedical Information

What other information is the orthopaedic surgeon likely to seek? Investing, travel, sports, and weather are the most popular topics. Weather is always of interest, especially when you travel. Look to **www.weather.com**. When you want information on travel go to **http://www.expedia.com** or **www.travelocity.com**.

There are many Web sites just to keep you current with digital imaging and photography. There are weekly newsletters that are sent to my e-mail box monthly to remind me to visit the Web site and read a new product review. Digital Photography Review is one of the best at **www.dpreview.com**. See also **http://www.pcphotoreview.com/**. To start your exploration of online photography go to **www.photo.net**. This is the largest collection of both online information about photography as well as 10,000 photographs. Registration is free. This site has lots to offer the beginner digital photographer.

For more information about traditional photography, visit the New York Institute of Photography (**www.nyip.com**). This site has archived a tutorial in digital photography that is of interest to both the beginner and advanced photographer. Online purchases of digital photography equipment can be made at **www.imagingspectrum.com** or **http://www.bhphotovideo.com/**—this is one of the largest warehouses of photo equipment in the US. If it is in stock, it ships out the next day.

If you want to compare your pictures with the best in the business, several professional photographers have posted their work on these sites:

www.dramainnature.com—spectacular light on landscapes,
www.soft.net.uk/pholio/—more extraordinary photos,
www.behindjackslens.com—galleries of photos,
www.karlgrobl.com—travel photos, and
http://www.altamira-group.com—photo galleries.

Reviewing the extraordinary composition of the images from these professionals always gives me inspiration and new ideas for my next photographic trip.

Books and music are the biggest sales from sites such as **www.amazon.com** and **www.ebay.com**. The latest sports scores can be accessed at *Sports Illustrated* (**http://sportsillustrated.cnn.com**). For news see *The New York Times* site (**www.nyt.com**), or *The Globe and Mail* (**www.globeandmail.com**).

Practical Tip. The handiest way to get the news, sports, and weather is to subscribe to multiple channels at Avantgo (**www.avantgo.com**). This information will be synched to your handheld PDA (Personal Digital Assistant) each morning. This way you don't have to go searching multiple sites to get the latest up-to-date information.

Other Information—The Good, the Bad, and the Ugly

Well, let's start with the ugly. If you have had an e-mail address for a few months, you know about the SPAM. Every day you receive free trips, one-in-a-million winner, university education, hot babes, Viagra, and on and on. This is the most annoying aspect of email. Even though you block the address today, they will send the same message tomorrow under a different name. Sex is a common search submission, so you know what sells. The Web content screening programs are essential for young children using the Internet, but not infallible. You have to have some discussion with your children about the potential X-rated Web pages that they will come across.

The aspects of the Internet that attracted the "early adopters" were the immense diversity of the information out there, the sense that we were part of an enormous change, the friendliness of the Internet, and the sense of community with colleagues half a world away. I belonged to several virtual communities: orthopaedics, photography, scuba diving, and natural history. My daughter as a teenager spent much of her free time on the Internet interacting with a group of people she never met. We kept a wary eye on her as she went through several messy stages of angst, betrayal, and self-doubt instigated by the group. We could never decide if it was good or bad, but she seemed to get through several necessary stages in virtual reality without actually being in danger of making serious physical mistakes. Latterly, the friendly informative character of the Internet seemed to be replaced by a frenetic commercialism in which everyone on or off the Orthopaedic part of the Internet seemed to be trying to buy or sell something. This was responsible for the caution and rejection that characterized the relationship between official orthopaedic organizations and some of the orthopaedic Internet pioneers. The milieu suggested that they were out to pick your pocket! Academics, for the most part, is overtly an unpaid activity. At the beginning of the Internet the atmosphere was one of friendly free exchange of information. We have been through a period of intense commercialism and hucksterism. We would hope that in the next stage the Internet will settle back to a steady growth in experience with the medium, and growth of the institutions that are needed to guide the quality of information on the Internet for the future.

4
Searching the Internet

Introduction

You could search the Internet by surfing from site to site, checking whether the information you need is on the site. With over 120 million domains to hand search in this fashion, it is likely your stamina and indeed your lifetime will not last long enough to make a sizable impression! Like so many words, "searching" in the context of the Internet has a new and restricted meaning. When you wish to find information on a computer system you have the option of defining the subject of interest and asking the system to examine its database to see if that subject is mentioned. If it is, that same system could produce a list of addresses of the files containing the desired information. Owing to the automatic nature of the process, every rock on the beach is turned over. Such searches are so much more productive than hand searching that we tend to use them exclusively and forget some vital things. The first is that the "beach" or field of rocks being turned is not limitless and is only a small fraction of the universe of information out there. The second is that an automatic search may only pick up exactly what it is asked for, so unless your definition is extremely precise some valuable information will be missed. In the context of the Internet, searching is at the same time enormously productive, intensely frustrating, and fraught with hidden limitations.

Difficulties of Searching

Anyone can search! The Internet has thousands of seductive ways, inviting you to "search" for the information you need. Implied in the invitation is the promise that the searching strategy will find it if it is there and the more subtle implication that if it isn't found it isn't in existence. For most searching situations these implications are simply not true. And, unless you are a geek and interested in the mechanics of searching, this isn't what you want; you want to *find* things and don't have any interest in the process of searching. But finding is successful searching, so this section is about refining your searching techniques.

The problems inherent in finding what you need are

- the information you need may not be on the Internet;
- the search engine does not search the whole Internet;
- the search strategy is not comprehensive enough to find what you want;
- useful information is buried in a welter of irrelevant, poor-quality pages;
- you are searching for a subject on which there is an overwhelming amount of information, and need to define your search more narrowly.

If you have done any searching via computer you have probably experienced these problems and difficulties at first hand. It can be frustrating because machines are very literal and utterly unable to read your mind. Just before you put your foot through the monitor it may be worth muttering this simple question: "What would this be like without computers?" If you are performing a literature search through the 4000 journals of MEDLINE, you know good and well what the answer would be. Without computers it couldn't be done. So no matter how frustrating your search may be, it is a thousand times quicker and more productive than you would ever achieve on your own.

Different Types of Search

Clinicians understand the distinction between specificity and sensitivity. Clinical tests that are specific are positive if and only if the disease is present; Staph aureus in the joint aspirate is a pretty specific test for septic arthritis. But it certainly isn't the only test, nor will it catch all cases. There will be some infections caused by other organisms and there will be some infections caused by Staph aureus in which the cultures will be negative. But it is specific. Argue what you will, if the joint aspirate is growing the organism, you had better believe it and act accordingly. In the same clinical setting C-reactive protein is quite sensitive. It is elevated in most infections. You may not know exactly which organism you are dealing with, and there may be conditions with a high titer without an infection, but your index of suspicion goes way up with the CRP and one is entitled to some degree of optimism if it is low.

When dealing with an Internet search it is important to know whether you wish sensitivity, trying to make sure you find all the places with information, or specificity, looking for the best and most relevant sites. So as you sit down to do a search, consider why you need the information. If you are hoping to write a comprehensive review of the subject, you may want to frame a sensitive search strategy. Whereas if you are looking for a few high-quality sources of information, you need a highly specific search strategy. For this you frequently need and cannot avoid using Boolean logic.

Boolean Logic

Any sophisticated search engine uses the Boolean logic terms OR, AND, and NOT in precise ways to expand or contract a search. In a nutshell the result is that OR is used to expand the search, AND to look at the overlapping portions between two searches, and NOT to exclude a portion of the search. See Figure 4.1.

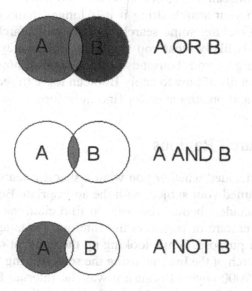

FIGURE 4.1. Examples of Boolean terms and their meanings

TABLE 4.1. Examples of Boolean terms and their meanings.

Boolean term	Means	Example	Means
AND	Together with	Hip AND Avascular Necrosis	AVN of the hip (only)
OR	Either/or	Osteonecrosis OR Avascular Necrosis	Either Osteonecrosis or Avascular Necrosis
NOT	Excluding	Avascular Necrosis NOT Hip	AVN of everywhere except the hip

Practical Tip. Use OR to expand the search, AND to look at the overlap, and NOT to exclude stuff.

A OR B means all of A, all of B including the overlap.
A AND B means only the overlap between A and B.
A NOT B means all of A except the overlap with B.

Note that some of the definitions in Table 4.1 are not intuitively what you might expect. If you search for Osteonecrosis AND Avascular Necrosis you might expect to get all the sites that refer to Osteonecrosis AND all the sites that refer to Avascular Necrosis. Instead you would get only those sites that refer to BOTH Osteonecrosis and AVN. To increase sensitivity you would use OR. To increase specificity you would use AND and NOT.

One of the concealed features of search engines is that they apply Boolean logic to your search string if it is longer than one word. If you search for Hip Fracture, some search engines will search for Hip AND Fracture (which is likely what you want) but others may search for Hip OR Fracture and give you thousands of pages on hip hop and geological fracture lines. Details of how to apply Boolean logic to searches are given later in the segment on strategies for finding information on the Internet.

Different Search Regions

Once you have decided whether you want a specific search or a sensitive one and have framed your subject with the appropriate Boolean logic, the next step is to decide whether you want to find citations in the scientific (orthopaedic) literature or pages on the Internet. Once again your target depends on your purpose. While looking up the concept of Boolean logic I undertook a search of the Internet using the search string "George Boole" and found over 9000 pages. Because it was the Internet I could read any that were still posted and was able to find the full text one of Boole's original papers. But I have to trust that the information is correct: the page I found purports to come from Trinity College, Dublin, and I have no easy way of finding out if that is true or if the page posted by a named academic in Trinity College is a correct transcription of Boole's paper. If I want information whose quality is not taken entirely on trust, I must use the scientific literature. At least it is reviewed and the reputation of the journal and the originating institution is on the line. A search in MED-LINE for "Boolean Logic" AND orthopaedics yields no citations. However, a search for "Boolean Logic" on its own yielded 16 papers in the MEDLINE database of which one was entitled "Automatic query formulations in information retrieval." This is obviously very close to my current interest but the text is inaccessible. I can read the abstract but would have to find the 1983 issue of the *Journal of the American Society for Information Science* to read the text.

Although they have converged and will converge to a far greater extent in the future, there are currently two domains of information on the Internet, citations to the scientific literature which you can trust but cannot read and the Internet free-for-all which you can read but. . . .

Literature Citations

Creating a reading list or a list of references to a particular subject is now much easier than it ever used to be. The institution that maintains the largest computer database of citations is the US National Library of Medicine (NLM) which goes back in the medical literature to 1967. Since 1880 the US Surgeon General's Office maintained a list of medical journals. *Indexus Medicus* was started in 1876 and the computerized list of citations (MEDLINE) was started in 1967. Until recently MEDLINE searches were only done by medical libraries and they had to pay for the privilege. In 1998 NLM responded to the pressure for universally accessible "free" information and produced the PubMed site (current address **http://www.ncbi.nlm.nih.gov/PubMed/**) which allows free and unrestricted searching of the MEDLINE database of citations. This glorious freedom comes with a few expected and some unexpected drawbacks.

- It takes training and practice to frame suitable searches of MEDLINE.
- Some journals are not part of MEDLINE.
- PubMed uses a sophisticated logical system to translate your search string into terms that the searching system can use most efficiently. If you don't know what it is, this logical system can work against you.
- For orthopaedic subjects the most you should expect for free is the abstract of the article. There are links to the full text articles on the jour-

nal sites, but in most instances you must be a subscriber or use PPV to access them.

As can be seen from the list of links on this subject, providing a tutorial on using PubMed is a popular Internet activity. The NLM itself provides a very comprehensive tutorial at **http://www.nlm.nih.gov/bsd/pubmed_ tutorial/m1001.html.** Many of the others are shorter and chattier. Most are written by librarians. The only one written for orthopaedic surgeons is on Orthogate at **http://guide.orthogate.com/workshops/search/default. htm** and this workshop was prepared specifically for this book.

Before going into any further details about the PubMed searching facility, it may be useful to explain how the MEDLINE citations database was created and is updated. When a new edition of a journal is published, the publishing house sends a copy to NLM. The initial index is done very quickly and the title of the paper, the names of the authors, the abstract, and the reference are added to the database. I imagine that one of the conditions of having a journal added to the MEDLINE database is that the index material must be sent to NLM in a specific electronic format that can be transferred directly to the database. These entries are searchable and are given a PubMed Identification number (PMID) and designated [PubMed in process].

The librarian staff at NLM then gets to work to identify the keywords that apply to the paper. These are selected from the specific NLM vocabulary of medical subject headings (MeSH Terms) (**http://www.ncbi. nlm.nih.gov/entrez/meshbrowser.cgi**). These terms are added to the full citation record as well as links to the Web sites of some of the journals. Once this is complete the notation [PubMed—Indexed for MEDLINE] is placed in the citation instead of "in process." Since the MEDLINE search engine partly relies on the use of MeSH terms, it is clear that the outcome of searches depends on the quality of the indexing done by the librarians.

Framing suitable searches on MEDLINE is a skill which until recently was confined to medical librarians. It is still a skill and they are still the resource to turn to if you wish your search to be as comprehensive and specific as possible. However, the database the medical librarian actually uses is available to you as well since the introduction of PubMed. So if you want to do it yourself, you can. To do it adequately you need to train yourself. It is necessary to do this semiformally by doing one of the many workshops and then practicing the skills quite frequently. It is not intuitive and it is doubtful that you could train yourself just by using the site. If you do that you will get results but you might very easily become discouraged by the overwhelming number of citations and the seeming lack of relevance. Worse, you may think you have obtained a comprehensive search when you haven't.

MEDLINE indexes about 4000 journals by a recent count. If you select only those journals whose primary subject is orthopaedics, hand surgery, or orthopaedic sports medicine, MEDLINE has 102. However, there are many other orthopaedic publications that are not listed in MEDLINE (e.g., the *Bulletin of the American Academy of Orthopaedic Surgeons*). So although a MEDLINE search is as comprehensive as technology can make it, it will not be completely comprehensive. The old-fashioned way of collecting citations from review articles is still of value.

In order to search the database efficiently PubMed "translates" the search string into a set of logical instructions. As an example I started a search about the value of hip protectors in preventing hip fracture. The search string entered was protection against hip fracture (Figure 4.2).

Note that only 56 citations have been found, so this is a small subset of the nearly 9000 citations about hip fractures. But the first citation demonstrates one of the problems. The words "protection" and "hip fractures" occur in the title but the subject of the article is obviously different from our area of interest. Clearly some form of translation has taken place but exactly what is not certain. Fortunately, the PubMed site will explain. If you click on the "Details" link after you have undertaken a search, the way the search engine has used your search string is made clear (Figure 4.3).

Citations will be selected if the word "protection" occurs in any field (Title, Author List, Abstract, or Keywords) AND (Boolean AND) either the MeSH term "Hip fractures" has been indexed with the paper OR (Boolean OR) the text contains the words "hip fracture."

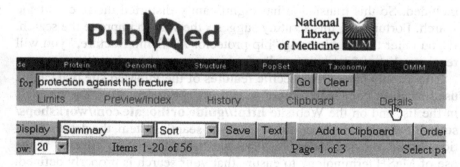

FIGURE 4.2. PubMed search for protection against hip fracture

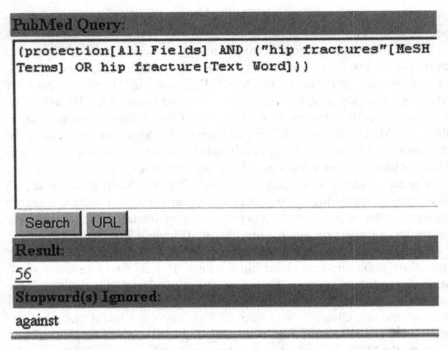

FIGURE 4.3. Details of the translation of the query, "Protection against hip fracture"

Note that the word "against" is ignored. There is a list of "stopwords" which occur so commonly that they would confuse the search if they were included. So this translation has significantly distorted the intent of the search. Fortunately, this scrutiny suggests the way to improve the search. If you enter the search string "hip protector AND hip fracture," you will receive a list of 23 citations, all of which are on the subject.

This is only one of the specific features of the PubMed site that can be used to make your search more specific or more sensitive. The tutorials in the list and on the Web site **http://guide.orthogate.com/workshops/ search/default.htm** cover use of the basic search system, the details function, limits, preview/index, history, and the cubby. Also covered is the use of MeSH terminology to ensure that your search is properly defined.

The point we have been attempting to make in this section is that searching MEDLINE through the PubMed interface is a very valuable skill that needs to be learned and practiced. We offer a number of links to teaching sites on PubMed.

Finding Orthopaedic Information on the Internet

Even if a search engine only has access to a fraction of the Internet, it does find over 300,000 pages that contain the word orthopaedic or orthopedic. Table 4.2 shows how additions of orthopaedic subject terms alter the number of pages found on the search engine AltaVista (**http://www. altavista.com**) (Sept. 2001). From the table we see that if we add the pages with the word "orthopaedic" on it to the pages with "orthopedic" (3), we get 295,000 pages. Adding "arthroplasty" (4) adds another 6000, which implies that there are 6000 pages with the word "arthroplasty" but *without* either of the words "orthopaedic" or "orthopaedic." Adding "sports medicine" (5) makes the number jump significantly, presumably because there are a lot of pages that mention sports medicine but make no mention of orthopaedics. Adding "fracture" (6) also makes the number increase, but we don't know if this is because a large number of nonorthopaedic sites talking about geology or metal fatigue are included. Row 7 is a search for pages that include either of the words "orthopaedic" or "orthopaedic" and at least one of the terms "arthroplasty," "fracture," or "sports medicine." This narrows it down considerably and (one assumes) eliminates pages that are about geology or orthopaedic mattresses. If a few more terms are added (8), we get a figure of more than 100,000 for the number of pages "about" orthopaedics in the AltaVista database. This is still a very poor estimate of the size of the Orthopaedic Internet since

- AltaVista only indexes a proportion of the pages on the Internet;
- there will be many pages that contain none of the search string terms which are about orthopaedics even so;

TABLE 4.2. The number of pages found by the Alta Vista Search Engine.

Search string with boolean term	Number of pages
1 Orthopedic	177,263
2 Orthopaedic	138,457
3 Orthopaedic OR Orthopedic	295,014
4 Orthopaedic OR Orthopedic OR Arthroplasty	301,248
5 Orthopaedic OR Orthopedic OR Arthroplasty OR "Sports Medicine"	466,711
6 Orthopaedic OR Orthopedic OR Arthroplasty OR "Sports Medicine" OR Fracture	705,248
7 (orthopedic or orthopaedic) AND (arthroplasty or "sports medicine" or fracture)	61,793
8 (orthopedic or orthopaedic) AND (arthroplasty or "sports medicine" or fracture or spine or hand)	111,365

- many of the pages indexed will be duplicates; and
- many of the pages found by this search strategy will not be mainly about orthopaedics.

Nevertheless the exercise does show that the Orthopaedic Internet is very large. And this has three corollaries: there is such a lot of stuff that there may well be some good stuff out there on a subject that interests you; finding the good stuff may be very difficult without a searching strategy; and no one, certainly not the authors of a book like this, knows all the best sites on the Orthopaedic Internet.

If you use a large library you have an idea of the strategies that are available to you when you want to look up something. You can find the library's copy of the best textbooks and look up the chapter on your subject. You can look through the catalog for titles on your subject. You can scan the table of contents of journals that you think may have articles about it. You can ask the librarian or in the last resort you can wander through the bookshelves hoping to find something. These strategies can be transferred to the Internet and correspond roughly to

visiting the textbook sites,
using an index site,
visiting the site of a journal,
using a search engine, and
random surfing.

Except for random surfing we examine each of these activities in detail. Don't, however, dismiss random surfing entirely. It is not an efficient way of finding something specific but it is still extremely likely that you will come across something interesting and valuable. Serendipity should not be ignored.

Textbooks/General Sites

Orthopaedics is extremely fortunate in having a resource of the size and quality of the *Wheeless' Textbook of Orthopaedics* (**http://www. medmedia.com**). Like many textbooks it originated as the notes of an orthopaedic trainee. C.R.Wheeless was a resident at Duke in 1996 and collected all his lecture notes and revision material into Web pages. Once these were linked and illustrated, the result was one of the first documents on the Internet to demonstrate the potential of hypertext as a form of academic expression. There have been many other erudite works of orthopaedic scholarship that have been posted on the Internet since, but nearly all have a textual basis and betray their origins as a piece of paper. Wheeless' achievement would be memorable if all he had done was to show that hypertext is different from text and that a hypertext document affords a journey through the information that may be unique to each visitor. However, he did more than that. His textbook is comprehensive, covering even the most abstruse subjects in orthopaedics with an introduction to the literature on the subject. The material betrays its origin as notes and its authorship by a person under instruction rather than an expert in the field. Since the original posting the site has been updated with numerous additions and improved illustrations. A number of guest authors and editors have been involved with the project.

One of the original aims of the Orthogate project was to incorporate *Wheeless' Textbook* into the site and continuously update it. This aim should perhaps be revisited as the Textbook, the Internet, and Orthogate mature. At present the Textbook is an outstanding resource for trainees and general practitioners and has much to offer experienced orthopaedic surgeons who are looking up an unusual subject. Because it has been on the Internet a comparatively long time it is well represented in the search engines and has been found by many patients. An AltaVista search shows that over 2200 other sites have links to *Wheeless' Textbook*. A well-informed, Internet-savvy patient who comes to your office may well have looked up their condition in *Wheeless' Textbook*—and be alarmingly well informed as a result.

World Ortho (**http://www.worldortho.com**) is another early arrival on the orthopaedic Internet that has provided an important resource to a large readership. The site is the work of the Orthopaedic Department at Nepean Hospital, Sydney, Australia, and features the cases and teaching material assembled at that institution, notably by R.L. Huckstep. The main resources of the site are Web versions of the textbooks and lecture notes written by Professor Huckstep and Dr. Eugene Sherry. These include

- A Simple Guide to Orthopaedics (PDF version) (**http://www. worldortho.com/database/sgo/index.html**);
- Typhoid Fever and Other Salmonella Infections (**http://www. worldortho.com/huckstep/typhoid/index.html**);
- World Ortho Electronic Textbook (**http://www.worldortho.com/ database/etext/index.html**);
- Lecture Notes (**http://www.worldortho.com/database/lectures/ lecture1.html**);
- Hot Topics (**http://www.worldortho.com/hot_topics/index.html**);
- A Photographic Tutorial on Musculoskeletal Examination (**http://www.worldortho.com/database/msexam/indexb.html**);
- A Simple Guide to Trauma (**http://www.worldortho.com/database/ sgt/index.html**);

- Core Orthopaedic Topics (**http://www.worldortho.com/core.html**). These include the Neuropathic Limb, Congenital Conditions, oliomyelitis, Tumors, Arthritis, Paralysis, Osteomyelitis
- Color Guide to Sports Medicine (**http://www.worldortho.com/sportsmed/cover.html**); and
- Oxford Handbook of Sports Medicine (**http://www.worldortho.com/oxsportsmed/index.html**).

World Ortho also has a number of teaching cases in quiz form, case presentations, and items on the history of orthopaedics. *Wheeless' Textbook* is also mirrored on the WorldOrtho site as is an early and obsolete version of OWL.

This site is a complete contrast to *Wheeless' Textbook*. There is an amazing amount of material collected and organized by leading experts. However, this material is imported from printed textbooks. A linear pattern is introduced as a result with little opportunity to digress, link to other resources, or look deeper into any subject. Much of the material is aimed at medical students, GPs, and residents. It is also a popular and widely connected site with about 1500 other pages linking to WorldOrtho.

A major undertaking in this area has been started by the Southern Orthopaedic Association under the title of the *Orthopaedic Care Textbook* (**http://www.orthotextbook.net/**). This offers to post a comprehensive, peer-reviewed, Internet textbook on orthopaedic surgery and related specialties. The site is currently accessed by use of a freely available password. This will change shortly when the password will only be available to readers of the *Journal of the Southern Orthopaedic Association.*

Each subject has a chapter written by named experts in the field and is quite structured with sections entitled Introduction, Historical Perspective, Anatomy and Physiology, Natural History, Diagnosis, Treatment, and Summary. There is also a patient information section that summarizes the chapter in nontechnical terms and a list of references with a link to the MEDLINE abstract. Also standard for each chapter are links to an outline of the chapter, pharmacology giving details of the medications mentioned, figures, and equipment. The equipment section has a discussion of the products described in the chapter with links to the suppliers' Web pages. Clearly, this is a well thought out and valuable resource. It remains to be seen how many of the subject headings will be covered.

Although they are not strictly textbooks, there are a number of review sites that qualify for this section. There is a reasonable chance of finding some coverage of the orthopaedic subject you are looking for on these sites. They have collected trainee's presentations or are aimed at orthopaedic trainees. Although some of these require a password, registration is otherwise free.

- South Australian Orthopaedic Registrars' Notebook, Flinders University of South Australia (**http://som.flinders.edu.au/FUSA/ ORTHOWEB/notebook/home.html**);
- OrthoNet (University of Toronto Residents' Site) (**http://orthonet. on.ca/mainpage.asp**);
- Orthoteer, Orthopaedic Study Syllabus (Ireland) (**http://www. orthoteers.co.uk/**); and
- Othopedics Hyperguide, preparation for the Fellowship exams; sponsored by Stryker (**http://www.ortho.hyperguides.com/**).

Index Sites

Another way to find information is to visit sites that provide lists of addresses to Web pages of orthopaedic interest. Yahoo (**http://www. yahoo.com**) was one of the earliest of this type of resource. However, since Yahoo tries to cover every subject on the Internet, its coverage of specific subjects is less comprehensive. There are also commercial concerns. You can pay the corporation to index a site. There are index sites maintained by libraries, and many institutions post a list of links on their Web pages. The most serious attempt to provide an index for the Orthopaedic Internet is Orthopaedic Web Links (OWL) (**http://owl.or- thogate.com**) which is edited by one of the authors of this book (Myles Clough). You will recall our estimate that the Orthopaedic Internet was larger, possibly much larger than 100,000 Web pages; Owl indexes 7000 pages.

The labor of collecting links and editing them into an index is enormous and it is not surprising that no index covers more than a tiny fraction of the Orthopaedic Internet. They do still provide certain advantages, the first being that someone has selected the sites as being of interest, presumably orthopaedic interest. OMNI (**http://omni.ac.uk**) has the most stringent inclusion criteria including evaluation by a reviewing committee. OWL is the selection over the last five years of a small group of orthopaedic surgeons. Sites that have an automatic inclusion process through a database program tend to have a predominance of commercial, institutional, and clinical Web sites with less emphasis on clinical and teaching material. A second advantage of these sites is serendipity. It is rare to browse through one of the index sites looking for a specific subject without coming across sites that are interesting enough to divert you. You may not count this an advantage if you are trying to remain focused!

TABLE 4.3. The size of Orthopaedic Index Sites (Sept. 2001).

Name and address	Number of orthopaedic links
OWL (http://owl.orthogate.com)	4000
Cliniweb Musculoskeletal Disease (http://www.ohsu.edu/cliniweb/C5/C5.html)	314
Cliniweb Wounds and Injuries (http://www.ohsu.edu/cliniweb/C21/C21.866.html)	170
Karolinska Institute Library Musculoskeletal Diseases (http://www.mic.ki.se/Diseases/c5.html)	548
Karolinska Institute Library Wounds and Injuries (http://www.mic.ki.se/Diseases/c21.html)	65
MEDLINE Plus Health Information (NLM) (http://www.nlm.nih.gov/medlineplus/ bonesjointsandmuscles.html)	1100
MedMark Orthopedics (http://medmark.org/os/os2.html)	ca. 900
DMOZ Open Directory (http://dmoz.org/Health/Medicine/Surgery/Orthopedics/)	378
Yahoo Orthopaedics (http://dir.yahoo.com/Health/Medicine/Orthopedics/)	64
Orthopaedics.com (http://www.orthopaedics.com)	434
OMNI Organising Medical Networked Information (http://omni.ac.uk)	353

Apart from the very incomplete coverage of the Internet, the main disadvantage of the index sites is "link rot." This is a colorful term for the process whereby the list of links gets out of date. Pages are withdrawn from the Internet and addresses are changed. Unless the Webmaster of the site doing this takes the trouble to notify the index sites, the links on those sites will be incorrect. The editor of the index page has to visit each site in the index at regular intervals and keep the links up to date. Without attention to this detail the index will be irritatingly misleading within six months.

Notifying the index sites of the posting of new material or updates will be a key issue for the future. Unlike publishing, there is no system (like MEDLINE) for indexing new contributions. It seems likely that one will evolve as the Internet matures and the quality of information is subjected to scrutiny. In fact the only workable mechanism for improving the quality of information on the Internet requires an index site of some sort. A clearinghouse, with a recognized authoritative index of the Orthopaedic Internet, to provide the most comprehensive and valuable service to the orthopaedic world, would be pivotal. Readers would naturally use it and pay attention to any comments made about the material. Those who post orthopaedic material would tend to notify the site in order to gain readership. This would put the index site in the position of being attended to when comments about the quality of the information on offer were made. Since you cannot and should not prevent people from posting Web pages, the only workable mechanism of quality control is to promote the readership of high-quality sites. Note that in this situation, competition between index sites is counterproductive. It would be a lot easier to know which site to use if one were predominant.

In 1995 OWL was consciously set up as a candidate for this pivotal role. There were two other groups with an interest in doing the same thing and all three merged in 1997. Although it is difficult to maintain the site and it has recently been transformed into a database, the need still exists and thus far there are no challengers as far as size and straight-to-the-meat content are concerned. OWL is by far the largest orthopaedic index (Table 4.3); it contains more links to orthopaedic patient information than the NLM's MEDLINE Plus and more links to commercial sites of orthopaedic supply corporations than the largest "Yellow Pages."

Search Engines

Search engines are specialized sites on the Internet that maintain a database containing the text of millions or thousands of millions of Web pages. When you wish to find the addresses of Web pages on a certain topic you can visit a search engine Web site and present it with a "search string" of words that define the topic of interest. The search engine analyzes the search string and then searches its database for all occurrences of these words. The search engine constructs some sort of relevance score based on the number of times the search string appears on the page. All Web sites in which the search string occurs are then presented, in order of "relevance." A page is constructed on-the-fly which has the title of the page, some relevant text, and a link. The result of a well-defined search request is a list of the sites on the Internet that most closely satisfy the request. However, it doesn't always work out like that.

The problems inherent in searching lie in the literalness and automatic nature of the process. If you ask for "orthopaedic," you will get everything with the word "orthopaedic" in it, including orthopaedic mattresses or orthopaedic-designed dance shoes! In fact, the Google Search Engine (**http://www.google.com**) will find 289,000 pages. It won't find pages with the word "orthopedic," and if you search for that term it will return 375,000 mostly different pages. In fact if you look at the first 10 found after each search, there is only one page (AAOS, **http://www.aaos.org**) appearing in both. So you can miss finding what you want by the simple problem of spelling.

Then there is the question of what do you do with 375,000 addresses. If you look at the first thousand, you still will find that most pages are about orthopaedics, clinics, university orthopaedic departments, or orthopaedic organizations. So the search isn't unsuccessful—it's too successful; it has produced such an overwhelming number of pages to choose from that you cannot use the results.

If you do a search for "arthritis of the hip," you will get a similarly large number of pages. But most of the pages in the first 100 are blatantly commercial, and information useful to you as an orthopaedic surgeon is hard to find. It is there, however. The 33rd page is **http://www.medmedia. com/o13/71191.htm,** the Hip Joint in Rheumatoid Arthritis from *Wheeless' Textbook,* and has a useful summary of the subject and a list of references. Also in the first hundred are

- Septic Arthritis of the Hip. Iowa Virtual Children's Hospital (**http:// www.vh.org/Providers/TeachingFiles/PAP/MSDiseases/ SepArthHip.html**);
- a posting of the abstracts of the American College of Rheumatology Conference with papers on the subject (**http://www.hopkins-arthritis.som.jhmi.edu/edu/acr2000/oa-epidemiology.html**);
- American College of Rheumatology Guidelines for Management of Hip Osteoarthritis (**http://www.rheumatology.org/research/ guidelines/guidelines/oa-hip/oa-hip.html**); and
- Radiology in Paediatric Emergency Medicine—a case study of septic arthritis of the hip (**http://www.hawaii.edu/medicine/ pediatrics/pemxray/v4c17.html**).

That's it for orthopaedic interest in the first 100 pages. All the rest are directed at patients (or pet owners). Some of the patient information pages are very useful (especially Dr. Huddlestone's Arthritis of the Hip and Knee Joint (**http://www.hipsandknees.com/**). But the general level is dismal. What complainers mean when they say that "there is no good stuff on the Internet" is that the pages most easily found are of poor quality. There is good information but you must search diligently and methodically to find it. We explain later why search engines tend to give prominence to commercial pages over scholastic and academic ones.

Another problem with searching is that you may not know what you are searching. Most search engines do not explain what database they are searching. They glibly say, "Search the Internet" as if they have access to everything that is currently posted. In fact most search engines "know about" only a fraction of the pages on the Internet. To demonstrate (Table

TABLE 4.4. The Number of pages found by different search engines (Sept. 2001).

Search engine	Hits for orthopaedic	Hits for osteolysis
AltaVista (**http://www.altavista.com/**)	243,945	2335
Excite (**http://www.excite.com/**)	17,365	65
HotBot (**http://hotbot.lycos.com/**)	138,200	2500
Yahoo (**http://www.yahoo.com/**) (Uses Google)	133,000	1280
Northern Light (**http://www.northernlight.com/**)	214,796	2634
Webcrawler (uses Excite)	17,365	1364
(**http://www.webcrawler.com/**)		
Google (**http://www.google.com/**)	238,000	4140
Netscape (**http://search.netscape.com**)	936	4
Look Smart (**http://www.looksmart.com**)	204	528
Lycos (**http://search.lycos.com**) (uses FAST)	157,863	3266
FAST (**http://www.alltheweb.com**)	193,800	3266

4.4), we reviewed the number of pages found by several different search engines looking at a very common search string, "orthopaedic," and a more abstruse one, "osteolysis."

Clearly each search engine searches a different subset of the Internet. Some of these subsets may even be sites that pay the search engine to promote their site. The problem is that we don't know what parts of the Internet they are searching. All one can say for sure from looking at the table is that there is wild variety between the search engines. Google stated it searched 1,610,476,000 Web pages. It is hard to estimate what proportion of the Internet that is. The number of hosts on the Internet grew from 213 in 1981 to 29,000,000 in January 1998 (*The Size and Growth Rate of the Internet* by K.G. Coffman and Andrew Odlysko, published by First Monday, 1998.) Current estimates can be obtained from **http://www. netsizer.com/index.html** and was 122 million in September 2001. This means that Google has about 10 pages per host in its database. Surely the average number of pages per host is 10 times that, which suggests that even the biggest search engines cover only a small fraction of the Internet. (See the article in *Wired,* **http://www.wired.com/news/business/ 0,1367,11448,00.html**) Search engines also do not search pages that are created on-the-fly from a database. You will not find any pages from PubMed through a search engine although you may find abstracts from the journal sites. This reinforces the artificial division between the Internet and "the literature."

A search often results in far too many sites to read. So you tend to look at only the first few. These sites should be the most relevant given the search engine's "relevancy" algorithm but they often seem to be the brashest. To understand this, we need to digress into the way that search engines "rate" sites.

A "search string" is a single word or group of words that you choose as a description of your subject of interest. When you enter a search string into a search engine it may come up with tens of thousands of pages where that search string is part of the text on the page. A site that would interest you may be there in the list but it would be unlikely that you have the stamina to look beyond the first few (perhaps the first 100 if you were really determined). So Web site designers recognize that to be "found" the site has to come up in the first dozen or so. Although each search engine is different and its relevancy algorithm is a trade secret, they all have one common feature: they rate the sites they index using an arithmetic process so that each site has a relevance score that relates it to your search string. The higher the score, the earlier in the list of Web sites the search engine will produce. What makes for a high score?

- The presence of the search string in the title of the page.
- The presence of the search string in the keyword list.
- The presence and frequency of the search string in the text on the page.
- The proportion of the text taken up by the words in the search string.

So to score highly the page should have the likely search string in the title, the keyword list, and the text but very little else. The more content there is on the page the more "diluted" the desired text will be and the lower the score. Canny Web page designers will thus produce a Splash Page which will have almost no text, so the attractiveness to search engines is maximized. On the AAOS home page (**http://www.aaos.org**) the only actual text is the address of the organization. All the rest is textual graphics which do not register with the search engines as text. The keywords placed on the site are "orthopaedic, orthopedic, surgery, surgeon, osteoarthritis, splinting, fracture, arthritis, joints, trauma, musculoskeletal, arthroscopy, total joint replacement, sports medicine, hip replacement, spine, knee, shoulder, elbow, foot, ankle, hand, knee replacement, tumor, cancer, infection, carpal tunnel, hip," so the Web designer has really covered the bases. It is also possible to pay some search engines to have a site come up early in specific searches. If you search for orthopaedic surgery on AltaVista, the AAOS site comes up eighth out of 2,235,635. This means that seven other Web site designers have done a better job of attracting that particular search engine. Creating a Web page that is so supremely attractive to search engines is a skill which doesn't come cheap. The top pages in most searches have spent money on their Web design. They either have deep pockets or they are trying to make money. Pages posted for the sake of informing orthopaedic surgeons often pay little attention to this aspect.

We researched this subject by searching for "orthopaedic surgery" OR "orthopedic surgery" in the following major search engines: Google (G), AltaVista (AV), Northern Light (NL), FAST (F), and Excite (E) (Table 4.5). Sites that did not respond were excluded. This table therefore gives us a view of the orthopaedic surgery sites that have been most successful in attracting the search engines.

Table 4.5 shows that very few sites appeal to all search engines. One gets the impression that AltaVista favors commercial sites and there is the question of whether these sites may have bought the privilege of turning up early in a search for orthopaedic surgery. Northern Light seems to value the number of times the search string turns up on the page and this results in an unusual collection. The collections posted by Google, FAST, and Excite had most in common, but only one site turned up in the first 10 for all three search engines.

One way to increase the value of your search is to use a so-called metasearch engine. These submit the search to several individual search engines and then collect and annotate the results. The "osteolyis" search was submitted to metasearch engines recommended by the Library and Information Technology Association (LITA) (**http://www.lita.org/committe/toptech/toolkit.htm**) and are shown in Table 4.6.

The reasons why using many of the metasearch engines returns smaller numbers of results than using single search engines is not explained. It may be that the engine requires a successful search from more than one of the constituent search engines.

In the last analysis successful use of the search engine depends on careful framing of the search string. There is a reward for specificity. If you submit the search string "avascular necrosis hip treatment" to Google, you get 2930 sites returned. Avascular necrosis of the hip and Legg Perthes are the principal subjects in the first 200 of these. The default connection between words in Google is AND, so this string is avascular AND necrosis and so on. If you add osteonecrosis, the search string becomes ("avascular necrosis" OR osteonecrosis) hip treatment and about 4500 sites are found. However, the number of sites that are principally about AVN is still the same (200). Learning to use the search engines successfully is a skill just like learning to use PubMed. We have prepared a workshop on the subject on the Web site (**http://guide.orthogate.com/workshops/search/find1.htm**) since it is difficult to learn this skill without being connected and having access to the search engines in question. One point to be considered is

TABLE 4.5. Orthopaedic surgery sites in the top
10 of 5 different search engines.

	Rank of appearance in				
Name of site with link	G	AV	NL	F	E
Internet Journal of Orthopedic Surgery and Related Subjects	9			4	6
American Board of Orthopaedic Surgery	1				3
Ortho Home Page	2			3	
AAOS American Academy of Orthopaedic Surgeons	3			2	
Dr. Zeman's Sports Medicine	8				1
Orthopedics Sites				9	8
Johns Hopkins Orthopaedic Surgery	4				
New York Orthopaedic Hospital	5				
University of Texas Southwestern Medical Center Dept. of Orthopaedic Surgery	6				
Orthopaedic Surgery on the Web	7				
Dept. of Orthopaedic Surgery, Indiana University	10				
AAOS—Your Orthopaedic Connection (Patient Information)		1			
Orthopaedic Surgeons of L.I., Assoc. Homepage		2			
Lake Tahoe Orthopaedic Institute		3			
Sun Valley Sports Medicine Home Page		4			
Minter Orthopaedics—Dr. Jon Minter—orthopaedic surgeon		5			
Norristown Orthopaedic Associates, Inc.		6			
Saskatchewan Physician Recruitment Project (SPRP)		7			
eurimed.com—European Internet Medical Community		8			
Weiss Orthopaedics		9			
Pennsylvania Orthopaedic Society		10			
MedicalAnswer.co . . . : Physicians : By Specialty : Orthopedic Surgery : Virginia (list of orthopaedic surgeons in Virginia)			1		
Orthopedic Surgery (Practice notice Gillette, Wyoming)			2		
Orthopedic Surgery (Albert Einstein College of Medicine)			3		
Orthopaedic Surgery Position			4		
Department of Orthopedic Surgery (South Hutzel Hospital)			5		
Clinic Search—Orthopedic Surgery (Las Vegas)			6		
Orthopaedics Orthopedic Surgery (Dubois Regional Medical Center)			7		
University of Minnesota Department of Orthopaedic Surgery			8		
Orthopedic Surgery Residency (McLaren Regional Medical Center)			9		
Orthopedic Surgery (St. Vincent's Surgery Center)			10		
Department of Orthopedic Surgery (Baylor University)				1	
Home Page (SICOT Société Internationale de Chirurgie Orthopédique et de Traumatologie)				5	

Name of site with link	Rank of appearance in				
	G	AV	NL	F	E
niigata_med_orthop_home_page (Japanese)				6	
Physician Assistants in Orthopedic Surgery—PAOS Unofficial Web site				7	
Orthopedic Surgery Forum				8	
Orthopaedic Surgery Center of Illinois				10	
Southern California Orthopedic Institute Home Page!					2
Orthopedic Surgery Residency Ring					4
ISOST—Home (Internet Society of Orthopaedic Surgery and Trauma)					5
U.A.B. Division of Orthopaedic Surgery, University of Alabama					7
Orthogate					9
Bone and Joint Sources					10

whether to look in several search engines or to get to know one very well. It certainly makes sense to get to know one site very well and to use it to refine the search string for maximum specificity and sensitivity. If you are still not satisfied with the pages you have found, it would be reasonable to use other search engines as well as the metasearch engines.

One caveat is to always be cautious about the time that you spend searching. The real problem is to start searching for one bit of information, get-

TABLE 4.6. Metasearch engines

Engine name and URL	Comments
Ixquick Metasearch (**http://www.ixquick.com/**)	Returned 3266 hits, the same number returned by FAST (single search engine)
Meteor (**http://www.meteor.com/**)	Purports to search 9 major search engines. Retrieved 27 pages on osteolysis
Vivismo (**http://vivisimo.com/**)	123 hits. The strategy of this site emphasizes relevance rather than a large number of hits
ProFusion (**http://www.profusion.com/**)	29 hits. High relevance
Fossick.com (**http://fossick.com/**)	104 results which maintained a high relevance
Metacrawler (**http://www.metacrawler.com/index_power.html**)	26 results

ting distracted, and winding up wasting an hour and never locating the original data. There are two search engines that only search orthopaedic sites, Orthoguide (**http://www.orthoguide.com**) and Orthosearch. At the moment Orthosearch is not available from its previous address (**http://www. orthosearch.com**), although it is accessible from WorldOrtho (**http:// worldortho.com/**). You can be sure that you will access orthopaedic sites if you use these search engines; unfortunately, the number of sites in their database is small. Orthoguide returned seven matches for osteonecrosis and Orthosearch returned 172, all from either the WorldOrtho site or from *Wheeless' Textbook.*

Journal Sites

Nearly all orthopaedic journals now have a Web site and many of them post their articles in full text format. Existing subscribers usually have free access to these pages but, increasingly, nonsubscribers can review the table of contents and can download specified articles for a fee (PPV). This fee is set much too high at the moment (often $25 US) but economic reality will soon lower the price as the journals realize that patients want to read their articles. 50 × $5 is more than 5 × $25! Since the cost to the journal is virtually zero as they are posting the pages anyway, we can expect market forces to exert their usual magic.

The point for those currently seeking orthopaedic information on the Internet is that you can browse the table of contents of most orthopaedic journals and in many cases can access the abstract for free. If you cannot do this from the journal site, you can from PubMed once you have found the article you think will help. The journal pages thus form an index site of a very special sort offering access to really high-quality information, albeit not in any defined order.

OWL has a list of journal sites at **http://owl.orthogate.com/publica. html.** Appendix 1 (Journals) also has a short list of journal sites associated with major orthopaedic organizations. PubMed has a function which produces a list of the recent contents of selected journals (**http://www. ncbi.nlm.nih.gov/entrez/jrbrowser.cgi**).

Finding What You Need

By the end of this chapter you may have come to realize that finding orthopaedic information on the Internet can be challenging. It's time to reassure you that the challenge can be met. It is worth meeting because there is good information out there (200 pages on AVN of the hip can't all be bad), because the patients are using this resource, and because the quality of information on the Internet will improve. Although it may not cover all eventualities, we offer the following pathway for finding what you need:

1. Define what you are looking for in as great detail as you can. Write a phrase or a sentence defining the information you wish to find. This might be "recent journal articles by Goodfellow on the outcomes of his unicompartmental knee replacement," or "whatever I can find about hip replacement in patients with osteopetrosis," or "the URL for Goodfellow's unicompartmental knee replacement supplier."

2. Revisit your phrase to see if you can make it more definitive using information from elsewhere. You may be able to find out that Goodfellow's unicompartmental knee replacement is called the Oxford knee or that Biomet supplies it. You can certainly define "recent" as after a certain date.

3. Review what you have written; decide whether you are going to search the literature or the Internet or both, and whether your search is to be for specific information or sensitive. Thus you will end up with four options: Specific Literature Search (Step 4), Sensitive Literature Search (Step 6), Specific Internet Search (Step 8), or Sensitive Internet Search (Step 10).

4. Specific Literature Search. Go to PubMed and enter as specific a search string as you can manage. If you enter (goodfellow[Author Name] AND unicompartmental[all fields]) AND ("1998"[PDat] : "2002"[PDat])), you will see three papers in which J.W. Goodfellow reports his results.

5. If not satisfied, broaden the search and then refine it as described in the PubMed tutorial: **http://guide.orthogate.com/workshops/search/ broad.htm.**

6. Sensitive Literature Search. Visit the PubMed site and enter your search string. It should be quite specific. Check through the list of citations until you find one that is on subject. Click the "Related Articles" link for that citation.

7. If not satisfied, broaden the search by adding to the search string using OR. Go back to Step 6.

8. Specific Internet Search. Use an index site. If unsuccessful, use a large volume search engine like Google. Use a highly specific search string and if unsuccessful delete some words.

9. If this doesn't work, use the techniques of sensitive search (Step 10) until you are sure that your target site is "caught," then increase the specificity.
10. Sensitive Internet Search. Define search string using synonyms with Boolean OR terms. Set the search engine to deliver 100 sites per page and then check out the tenth page. If most of the sites are still relevant, you can assume you will have over 1000 sites to visit.
11. If much of what you get is not relevant, refine the search string to exclude irrelevant material (e.g., NOT veterinary).
12. If you are not satisfied with the collection, visit several other search engines and metasearch engines.
13. If you are still not sure you have all the sites, then go through the OWL index and other large index sites.

Internet Bibliography

- Eight Internet Search Engines Compared 1997 (**http://www.firstmonday.dk/issues/issue2_2/peterson/**)
- Search Engine Sizes (**http://searchenginewatch.com/reports/sizes.html**) August 2001
- The Major Search Engines and Directories (**http://searchenginewatch.com/links/Major_Search_Engines/The_Major_Search_Engines/index.html**)
- The Calculus of Logic George Boole 1848 (**http://www.maths.tcd.ie/pub/HistMath/People/Boole/CalcLogic/CalcLogic.html**)
- George Boole (**http://www-groups.dcs.st-andrews.ac.uk/~history/Mathematicians/Boole.html**)
- Automatic query formulations in information retrieval: Salton G, Buckley C, Fox EA. *J Am Soc Inf Sci* 1983 Jul;34(4):262–80 (**http://www.ncbi.nlm.nih.gov/entrez/query.fcgi?cmd=Retrieve&db=PubMed&list_uids=10299297&dopt=Abstract**)
- *PubMed* from National Library of Medicine 2001 (**http://www.ncbi.nlm.nih.gov/PubMed/**)
- *Medical Subject Heading (MeSH) Browser* from National Library of Medicine 2001 (**http://www.ncbi.nlm.nih.gov/entrez/meshbrowser.cgi**)
- *PubMed Tutorial* from National Library of Medicine 2001 (**http://www.nlm.nih.gov/bsd/pubmed_tutorial/m1001.html**)
- *Step-by-step guide to searching PubMed:* Glenfield Medical Library, Sept. 2000
- *PCPA: INTERNET MENTAL HEALTH RESOURCES: PubMed Tutorial,* Pennsylvania Community Providers Association, Oct. 1999

- *Searching the New PubMed,* State University of New York Dept. of Optometry, July 2000
- *PubMed* Tutorial, University of Medicine and Dentistry of New Jersey (**http://www.umdnj.edu/librweb/newarklib/infed/ PubMedtutorial/index.html**)
- *Understanding Medical Subject Headings (MeSH®),* McGill University Health Sciences Library
- *Boolean Logic* (as applied to MEDLINE Searches), McGill University Health Sciences Library (2001) (**http://www.health.library. mcgill.ca/eguides/boolean.htm**)
- *WelchWeb: Searching MEDLINE with PubMed,* Johns Hopkins, 2001 (**http://www.welch.jhu.edu/help/guides/dbs/wpubmed.html**)
- *PubMed Tutorial,* Houston Academy of Medicine, July 2001 (**http:// www.library.tmc.edu/newpubmed.html**)
- *PubMed Review,* Ruth Lilly Medical Library Indianapolis, Feb. 2001 (**http://www.medlib.iupui.edu/ref/pubmed.html**)
- *Introduction to PubMed,* New York Academy of Medicine, 2001 (**http://www.nyam.org/library/training/handouts/pubmed.html**)
- *PubMed Additional Useful Features,* New York Academy of Medicine, 2001 (**http://www.nyam.org/library/training/handouts/ pubmedadd.html**)
- *Introduction to Medical Subject Headings (MeSH),* New York Academy of Medicine, 2001 (**http://www.nyam.org/library/training/ handouts/meshhandout.html**)
- *Quick Guide to Searching PubMed,* Memorial University of Newfoundland, July 2001 (**http://www.med.mun.ca/hsl/guides/ pmedgde.htm**)
- *PubMed Clinical Filters,* Yale University Medical Library, May 2001 (**http://info.med.yale.edu/library/reference/publications/pubmed/**)
- *PubMed,* D. Samuel Gottesman Library, Albert Einstein College of Medicine of Yeshiva University (**http://library.aecom.yu.edu/ databases/Pubmed.htm**)
- *PubMed Tutorial Menu,* Dalhousie, Halifax NS, 2001 (**http://www. library.dal.ca/kellogg/guides/pubmed/introlft.htm**)
- *New Improved PubMed,* University of Alabama, May/June 2000 (**http://www.uab.edu/lister/letter/0003new.htm**)
- *PubMed Database Tips,* University of Kansas School of Medicine—Wichita, April 2001 (**http://wichita.kumc.edu/library/pmtips. html**)
- *PubMed Tutorial,* University of Florida, Health Science Center Libraries, July 2001 (**http://www.library.health.ufl.edu/pubmed/ pubmed2/**)

- *Searching MedLine via PubMed,* Vanderbilt University Medical Center (**http://www.mc.vanderbilt.edu/tutorial/tutorial_toc. html?tutorialID=3**)
- *PubMed Tipsheet,* University of Kansas Medical Center (**http:// library.kumc.edu/tipsheets/electronic/pubmed.htm**)
- *PubMed,* California State University of Long Beach (**http://www. csulb.edu/library/instruction/handouts/PubMed.html**)
- *The Spider's Apprentice — How to use Web Search engines,* Monash University. 2001 (**http://www.monash.com/spidap3.html**)
- *Search Engines & other miscellaneous links*, Dept. of Orthopaedic Surgery, Louisiana State University Health Sciences Center at Shreveport (**http://www.ortho.lsumc.edu/Geo/NBLinks.html**)
- *All Search Engines are not Created Equal, Wired Business News*, April 2001 (**http://www.wired.com/news/business/0,1367,11448, 00.html**)
- *AAOS Website,* American Academy of Orthopaedic Surgeons (**http:// www.aaos.org**)
- *Wheeless' Textbook of Orthopaedics,* 1996–2001 (**http://www. medmedia.com**)
- *WorldOrtho* Nepean Hospital, Sydney, Australia, 1996–2001 (**http:// www.worldortho.com**)
  - *Orthopaedic Care Textbook,* Southern Orthopaedic Association, 2001 (**http://www.orthotextbook.net/**)
  - *South Australian Orthopaedic Registrars' Notebook*, Flinders University of South Australia (**http://som.flinders.edu.au/FUSA/ ORTHOWEB/notebook/home.html**)
  - *OrthoNet* (University of Toronto Residents' Site) (**http:// orthonet.on.ca/mainpage.asp**)
  - *Orthoteer*, Orthopaedic Study Syllabus (Ireland) (**http://www. orthoteers.co.uk/**)
- *Othopedics Hyperguide,* Preparation for the Fellowship exams, sponsored by Stryker (**http://www.ortho.hyperguides.com/**)
- *OWL Orthopaedic Web Links,* 1996–2001 (**http://owl.orthogate.com**)
- *Cliniweb Musculoskeletal Disease,* Oregon Health Sciences University (**http://www.ohsu.edu/cliniweb/C5/C5.html**)
- *Cliniweb Wounds and Injuries,* Oregon Health Sciences University (**http://www.ohsu.edu/cliniweb/C21/C21.866.html**)
- *Karolinska Institute Library Musculoskeletal Diseases* (**http://www. mic.ki.se/Diseases/c5.html**)
- *Karolinska Institute Library Wounds and Injuries* (**http://www. mic.ki.se/Diseases/c21.html**)

- *MEDLINE Plus Health Information* (NLM) (**http://www.nlm.nih. gov/medlineplus/bonesjointsandmuscles.html**)
- *MedMark Orthopedics* (**http://medmark.org/os/os2.html**)
- *DMOZ Open Directory* (**http://dmoz.org/Health/Medicine/ Surgery/Orthopedics/**)
- *Yahoo Orthopaedics* (**http://dir.yahoo.com/Health/Medicine/ Orthopedics/**)
- *Orthopaedics.com* (**http://www.orthopaedics.com**)

5
Internet Applications

E-Mail

E-mail has become one of the most popular uses of the Internet. It is simply a method of sending messages from one computer to another. It does not have to use the Internet, but can use an intranet or a local area network connecting two business computers. An e-mail program is a word processor that uses the point of presence (pop) protocol to connect to the other computer. There are several different popular e-mail programs—Outlook, Outlook Express, AOL, MSN, and Eudora—but they are all very similar.

How do you get started? You need to have an Internet connection and an e-mail box. If you signed on with AOL or MSN, an e-mail address will be set up for you. If you have local ISP, it will give you a local phone number to dial, or configure a high-speed cable modem or high-speed

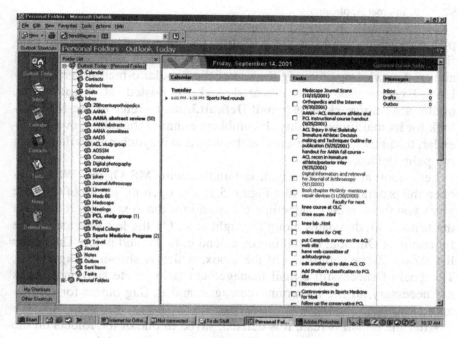

FIGURE 5.1. The opening screen of Outlook

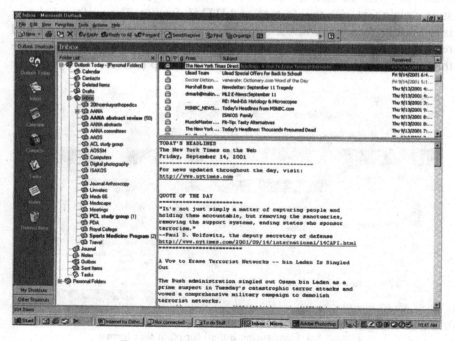

FIGURE 5.2. The e-mail in-box of Outlook

phone modem. Again the ISP will give you an e-mail address and configure this to work in one of the e-mail programs such as those mentioned above. A workshop covering the use of the popular e-mail program Outlook Express has been prepared and is posted at **http://guide.orthogate.com/workshops/email/Default.htm.** I prefer to use MS Outlook for its multifunctionality. It combines e-mail, scheduling, events calendar, to-do lists, messages, and addresses, and it synchronizes daily with my palm device.

Let's look at Outlook, which is bundled with MS Office. When you open the program it looks like Figure 5.1. The opening screen of Outlook gives you those events happening today and for the next week. It displays the tasks, with due dates along the right side. On the left side are all the functions of Outlook: e-mail inbox, calendar, tasks, and notes. The folder list shows all the subfolders of the inbox, which is shown in Figure 5.2. The goal of successful e-mail management is to delete anything that is not necessary, to file important messages, and to flag others for follow-up action.

After the e-mail is read, it is deleted, saved in one of the folders on the left, or flagged for later action. This keeps the current inbox to a manageable size. First, let's customize the software. Under tools, select options, and mail format, as shown in Figure 5.3. There are usually three styles: plain text, rich text format, and HTML format. The preferred choice is to use the plain text without formatting. Most other e-mail programs will read this easily. If you need to send a formatted MS Word document, use the attachment; it looks like a paper clip on the top toolbar. Now you have

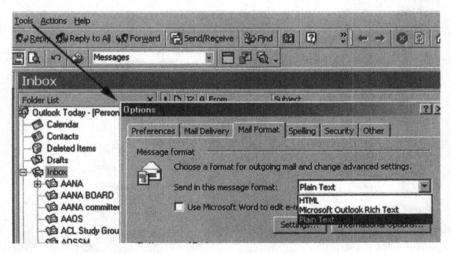

FIGURE 5.3. Configuring e-mail for plain text format

to know where the attachment is stored on your hard drive. Once you find it, it can be attached to the outgoing e-mail message. Remember, for the speed of transmission, keep the size of attachments to less than 200 Kb. Many e-mail servers have a maximum size for files, usually 1 Mb, and have a maximum size for the mailbox, frequently 2 Mb. This size limitation may be changed in the e-mail program or by making suitable arrangements with the ISP. For the Outlook Express Workshop on setting up, see **http:// guide.orthogate.com/workshops/email/setup.html.**

Sending a New Message

To send an e-mail, click on the inbox, select "new message," type in the address or select the recipient from the address book, state a subject, type the message, and hit the send button. Inserting e-mail addresses takes a little time. You have to enter all your contacts, their phone numbers, office and home phones, and the e-mail address. This requires a lot of typing. This is something that you should contract out to a secretary with good typing skills. One of the easy ways to add new contacts is from the e-mail address that comes when someone sends you a message. This can be clicked on and added to your address book.

The message is then routed in packets via many computers to the address requested. The messages usually arrive in seconds, but sometimes will get diverted for several hours. It is remarkably reliable, but unless the receiver acknowledges that he has received the message, you may never know if the message was actually delivered. If the message is important, you can request acknowledgment of receipt of the message. The receiver can reply, forward, print, or delete your message. (For the Outlook Express workshop on sending e-mail messages, see **http://guide. orthogate.com/workshops/email/send.html.**) So, that looks simple, but let's go into a little more detail on the e-mail programs.

In the address book, you can set up group mailings to committee members. This works well for communicating with all the members of a committee by sending out only one message. This is configured in the address book by picking "new group" and adding members from your address book to the group. See Figure 5.4.

Using the PDA also makes adding contacts painless. When you want to add another Palm user's information, the other Palm can send all its information to your Palm with infrared transfer by one click on the address book icon. However, after an annual professional meeting, you still are faced with entering data by hand from business cards. For the workshop on the Outlook Express address book function, see **http://guide. orthogate.com/workshops/email/addrssexp1.html.**

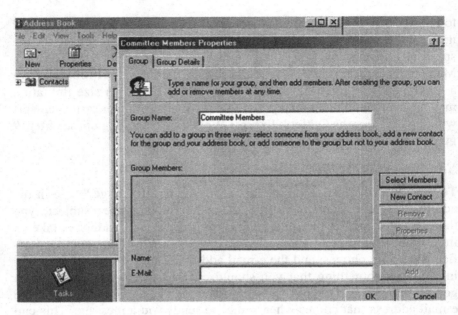

FIGURE 5.4. Setting up a new group by adding members from your address book

This is one more reminder about backing up data. The address and phone number information is stored in the Outlook folder on your computer. The backup file can be made by going to file, import and export. Select the export to a file, select personal folder .pst, and then select the folders that you would like backed up and where you want the file sent. Now you have all the important information stored somewhere else. There are also Internet-based programs that will store the data from your laptop, desktop, Palm, and phone all at one site. This is one of the most secure ways to back up. If you are out of town, and have a problem with your computer, you can still access the site and get the information that you stored there. It also makes sense to store important presentations on an Internet site such as **www.fusionone.com**.

Once you have selected the proper e-mail address for the recipient, you need to enter a subject. When the message arrives in the other mailbox, the only two pieces of information that are displayed are the sender's name and the subject. If you get a lot of e-mails daily, many are deleted at this stage. If you don't know the sender and the subject does not interest you, hit the delete button. A window will appear to confirm if you want to delete the message and you press enter to remove the message from your inbox. If later you want to view the message, you can go to the deleted box and read the message. Also at this stage, you can tell if there is an attachment. Usually a paper clip icon will be attached to the message. If you are unsure of the sender, and the subject is something like "important message," or the word "love" in any form, chances are it is a virus. Even if you are sure of the sender you may be receiving a virus if his or her e-mail address book has been infected. Many viruses are sent through the Outlook e-mail address book. You may get a message with an attachment from someone you know, who has been infected with a virus. The virus is transmitted via the attachment, but only causes damage when you are curious and open the file. Don't open any suspicious e-mail attachments. At the present time the virus will only affect your system if you open the attachment. For further information about viruses, see **http:// guide.orthogate.com/workshops/email/antivirus.html,** and for specific treatment of e-mail viruses and hoaxes, see **http://guide.orthogate.com/ workshops/email/antivirus2.html.**

Internet-Based E-Mail Programs

One of the significant advantages of using an Internet-based e-mail program such as Hotmail is the automatic virus scanning. Hotmail is the free

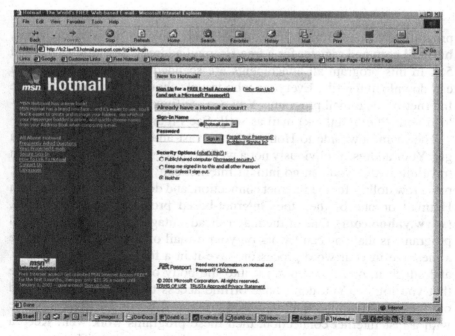

FIGURE 5.5. The opening registration screen for free Hotmail

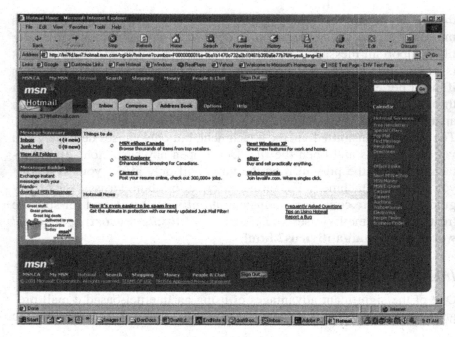

FIGURE 5.6. The Hotmail opening screen

program provided from Microsoft. All you have to do is go to **www. hotmail.com** and register for a free Hotmail address. See Figures 5.5 and 5.6. In this program all attachments are scanned for viruses before you can download the file. Everyone who travels should have one of the free Internet-based e-mail programs. You can configure the program to download your POP (Outlook) mail as well. See Figures 5.7 and 5.8.

The main downside to Hotmail is the vast amount of SPAM that you get. Your address is obviously not a well-kept secret. The advantage when traveling is that you can go into an Internet café anywhere in the world, pay a few dollars for the Internet connection, and do all your e-mail through Hotmail or one of the other Internet-based programs such as Yahoo, (**www.yahoo.com**). One of the major disadvantages of the Internet-based programs is that you can't work on your e-mail offline. You have to type a message in your word processor, save it in a folder on the hard drive, and attach it, or cut and paste it into the body of the text the next time that you log on. You don't have offline access to the address book and old messages with the Internet-based programs. If you are always online with a fast Internet connection, then these programs work well. Keep a printed list of your address book if you use these programs. That way you can access the information offline.

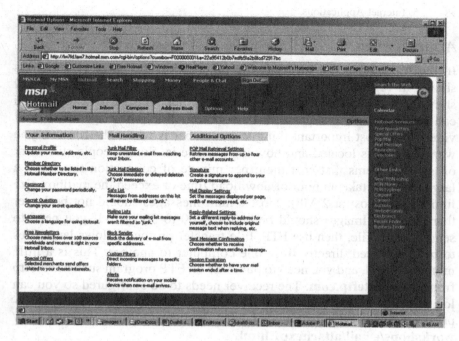

FIGURE 5.7. Configuration of Hotmail to download your POP e-mail messages

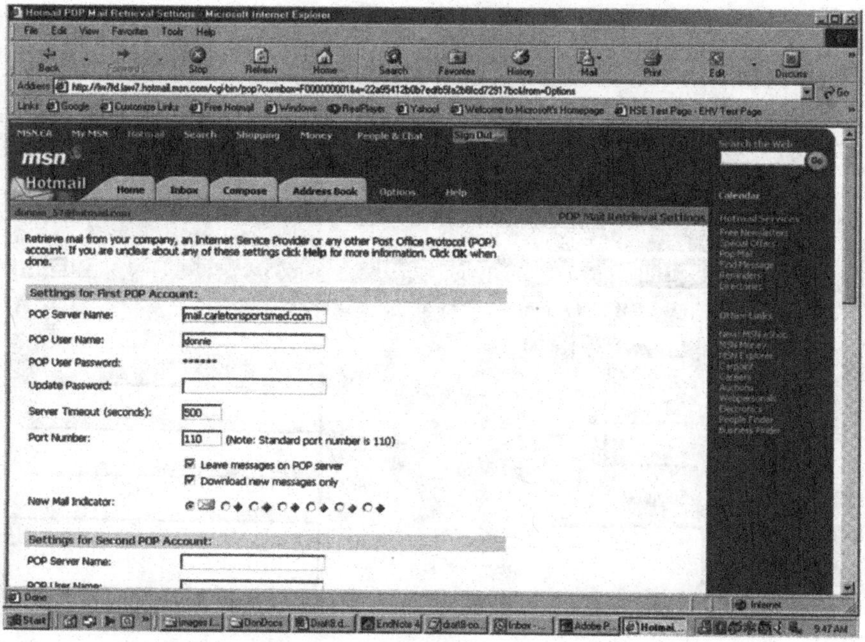

FIGURE 5.8. The second screen to enter your POP information

Attachments

In the top toolbar, go to insert file or click on the paper clip icon as shown in Figure 5.9. When you click on this, an explore function will show your hard drive. In the appropriate folder on the hard drive, you can select a word document, a PowerPoint slide, an image, or a short video. The most important thing to remember is where the file that you want to send is located and how big the file is. Some people still work on slow modems that cost them per minute of connection time, and a large file may take an hour of download time or exceed the mailbox size limitations (most at 2 Mb). Most e-mail messages should not be larger than 200 Kb. Images should be kept to 200 to 300 Kb. If you need to send a larger file, then use FTP. File transfer protocol allows large files to be transferred directly from one computer to another. This is a little more technical, and you need to purchase an FTP program such as cuteftp from **www.cuteftp.com**. The receiver needs to be configured so you can log into the other computer to allow the transfer. For the Outlook Express workshop on e-mail attachments, see **http://guide.orthogate.com/workshops/email/attachexp1.html.**

For short messages, instead of an attachment, copy and paste the text into the body of your e-mail message. If you are using the text-only ver-

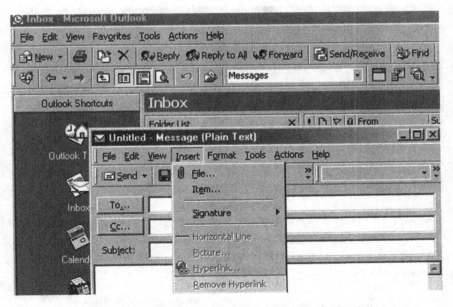

FIGURE 5.9. Inserting an attachment to an e-mail message

sion of the e-mail program, you are sure to have the message be readable. There are still configuration problems between e-mail programs, Word and Word Perfect, and PC and Macs.

Replying to an E-Mail Message

When you receive an e-mail message, you can hit the reply button and send a message back to the sender. You can configure your e-mail program to include the original message if this is important to the discussion. If it is not, delete the original message and just send the reply. This keeps the amount of data moving around to a minimum. When you send the reply, you can copy the message to other members of your address book. You can forward the message to other e-mail addresses and copy anyone in your address book. You can send copies to the significant others who should be included in the discussion. It is often better to use the bcc rather than the cc option. The bcc will not display the names and addresses to the people you have copied. Of course if you want everyone to know who was copied, use the cc function. The "reply to all" will send the return message to everyone who is on the cc list.

When a message arrives and it needs a more detailed response, you can flag the message for later attention. The message then sits on top of all the other messages with a red flag to draw your attention to it. If this needs a longer document composed, it can be done offline and attached to the reply that will be sent the next time that you log on. The Outlook Express workshop on replying and forwarding is at **http://guide.orthogate.com/workshops/email/replyexp1.html.**

Forward Message

This functions in much the same way as the reply to, but you can send the e-mail directly to another person for his or her information. The difference with reply is that you do not have to select a recipient address, and with forward you have to select the recipient. You can add your comments in the body of the message in the same way as with the reply to function.

Delete Message

This is my favorite button. You can often tell from the subject line that you have no interest in the message. Likely messages to delete include obvious advertisements, get rich quick offers, and ones from people you detest! Senders of SPAM often have e-mail addresses with numbers in them. The combination of numbers and a multiple outlet domain name like abc123@msn.com is a giveaway. Be particularly careful if there is an e-mail attachment as that is how most of the viruses are spread by e-mail. You should hit the delete button if you don't recognize the sender of the e-mail attachment. Remember that hitting delete will not, in fact, completely eliminate the message. It is still there in your "Delete" folder. This is good and bad. Good in that you can get back something you deleted by mistake and bad in that the dangerous virus code in the message is not eliminated and won't even be overwritten on your hard drive until after you empty the delete folder. I try to remember to empty the e-mail delete file every day. Outlook can be set to automatically empty the deleted files when you exit the program as shown in Figure 5.10.

Several of the viruses will go to your address book and replicate to everyone on your address list. The next day it then wreaks havoc on your hard drive. The body of the message often gives it away: "This file is the one requested." Don't open the file, even if it is from someone you know. If you are in their e-mail address book, the virus is being sent to everyone in their book without his or her knowledge. The message that caught me last week was entitled "Microsoft case settlement details." Fortunately, McAfee, my antivirus program, was smarter than I was and warned me not to open it and to do a complete scan of my system. Keep your e-mail

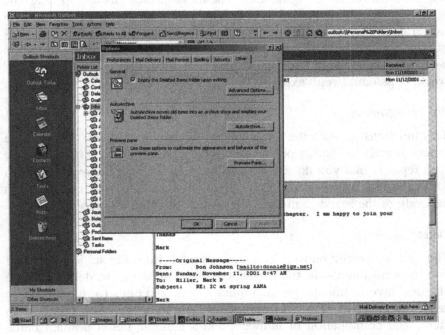

FIGURE 5.10. Setting Outlook to empty the deleted files automatically

and antivirus programs updated regularly. One recent virus took advantage of the "preview pane" in the Outlook e-mail program. This allows you to see the text of the message without formally opening it. If the preview pane is open, simply clicking on the suspect message to select it for deletion will open it in the preview pane. Even though you didn't fully open the message or its attachment the virus could infect your system. This vulnerability was halted by an update of the e-mail program; but, of course, if you don't update you may still be vulnerable.

Practical Tip. If you see a message with an attachment that you are not expecting, close the preview pane and put it in a special "suspect" folder without opening it (see below). If you know who sent it, send him or her a message asking what was in the attachment. If you are not satisfied, you can delete the message later. It won't harm you unless it is opened.

E-Mail Folders

One of the main features of Outlook is keeping all the e-mail messages organized. Important e-mails may be assigned to separate folders (I have about 30 folders) in the inbox. To set up a new folder, open the inbox folder list. If the folder list is not visible on the left side, go to the view menu on the top bar and click on the folder list. Under the folder list are calendar, contacts, deleted items, drafts, and inbox, as shown in Figure 5.11.. Right click on the inbox and select the new folder icon. The prompt window will ask for a name for this new folder and where you would like to put it.

Now all the items that pertain to that subject can be removed from the inbox and dropped into the folder. An empty e-mail box is an optimal but seldom achieved goal. It is impossible to wade through hundreds of messages to try to find an old message that was important (although there is a "Find" facility under the edit menu). These important e-mails may also be dropped on your "to-do" list and a time and date for action can be assigned. This same e-mail can be dropped into the calendar and a new event can be assigned.. Each morning the Outlook for the day is examined and the information is transferred to the PDA with the synchronization function. Since I carry my PDA around all day and check it regularly, I should not overlook any important meetings or calls. Outlook may have a little longer learning curve, but if your life consists of a lot of meetings, timelines for projects, to-do lists, and complicated scheduling, then Outlook does all these tasks well. The subject of folders in Outlook Express is posted at **http://guide.orthogate.com/workshops/email/foldrexp1.html.**

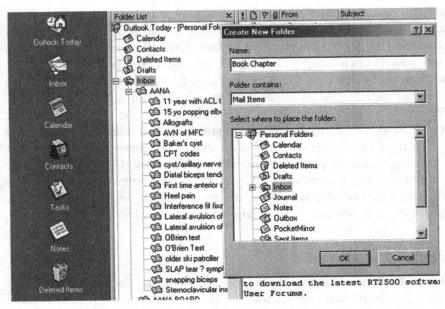

FIGURE 5.11. Setting up a new folder

Virus Hoaxes and Urban Legends

A common entertainment for a certain section of the population was to start a rumor usually predicting some dire event, and send it off by e-mail into cyberspace with exhortations to send this to everyone on your list of contacts. Virus hoaxes were particularly common. One assumes that the payoff for the instigators of these hoaxes was to see their creations flying by on the wings of panic and ignorance.

The urban legends were more inventive but some were cruel. I heard of one linking use of antiperspirant to breast cancer, which was causing a lot of anxiety at the hospital. The hallmark of these fabrications was that they were attention grabbing and had that tinge of credibility that made people likely to pass them on.

One well-crafted virus hoax urged you to examine your system files for evidence of "undetectable" virus infection and to delete certain named files if they were found. Trouble was that everyone using WINDOWS™ has these files, which are an integral part of the operating system. People who followed the instructions on the virus hoax message did themselves a significant mischief.

It is not completely safe to assume that any dire warning is a hoax but it is much more likely than not. The only thing that we can do to reduce the nuisance is to check out the rumors. This should certainly be done if you are contemplating actually sending on the message. These hoaxes are so common that there are well-organized sites collecting information about them—check on one of these sites to match your message against a known hoax:

Hoaxbusters, part of the Computer Incident Advisory Capability of the US Dept. of Energy (**http://hoaxbusters.ciac.org/**),
Internet Scambusters™ (**http://www.scambusters.org/**),
Norton AntiVirus Page on Hoaxes (**http://www.symantec.com/avcenter/ hoax.html**), and
Vmyths.com (**http://www.vmyths.com/**).

This subject is also reviewed at **http://guide.orthogate.com/workshops/ email/antivirus2.html.**

Practical Tip. Don't pass on warnings without checking. Don't open or download attachments from someone you don't know. Don't open attachments that look suspicious.

Mailing Lists, Bulletin Boards, and Discussion Groups

What are mailing lists? A mailing list is a collection of e-mail addresses that can be used to simultaneously send out a message to everyone on the list. Usually the people on the list will have a similar interest and a few will reply to the message and that reply is again distributed to everyone. This process is called a thread. These messages can be automatically archived for those who want to review the entire discussion at a later date. Examples of mailing list archives are found at

Orthopod Archives—**http://www.orthogate.com/cgi-bin/ezmlm-cgi/0,**
Hand Archives—**http://www.orthogate.com/cgi-bin/ezmlm-cgi/1,**
Sports Medicine Archives—**http://www.orthogate.com/cgi-bin/ ezmlm-cgi/4,**
Spine Archives—**http://www.orthogate.com/cgi-bin/ezmlm-cgi/2,** and
Arthroplasty Archives—**http://www.orthogate.com/cgi-bin/ezmlm-cgi/3.**

Mailing lists allow us to share information about a clinical problem with colleagues who have similar interests. The patient information, including X-ray images, can be posted, and similar to a presentation at rounds, several comments will usually follow. Be careful to guard the patient's confidentiality when posting X-rays.

How Do Mailing Lists Work?

Usually an organization will have all the members' e-mail addresses in one database. This can be automatically managed by a computer list server to post messages to everyone on the list. New members may join by sending a message to the computer to join the list. Newbies should learn the netiquette of the list, by listening in for the first few times. Learn that typing in capitals is equivalent to SHOUTING, learn not to be overly critical, and learn not to overtly advertise your wares or promote yourself. There are many other conventions that you will learn over time.

Examples of the mailing lists are:

Orthopod—a general orthopaedic mailing list,
Hand—a list exclusively for hand discussion,
Arthroplasty—a list for discussion of arthroplasty,
Spine—a list to discuss spinal problems, and
Sports Medicine—a discussion list of sports medicine topics.

The instructions to sign up for these mailing lists are on this page: **http://www.orthogate.com/modules.php?op=modload&name=EZCMS&file=index &menu=5&page_id=4.** For example, to join the "orthopod" mailing list send a blank e-mail message to **orthopod-subscribe@orthogate.com.** The message must be sent from the address you wish to have as the mailing list address, that is from your own computer or from your Hotmail account if that is how you want to set it up.

Practical Tip. Join a mailing list, but save the instructions about how to subscribe, and especially how to get off the list. After two weeks you may find that you have hooked up with the wrong crowd, and now want to get out but have deleted the instructions. Don't send, "I want to unsubscribe" messages to the list, as this message goes out to everyone on the list. The address to cancel the subscription is different.

For more information about orthopaedic mailing lists, see **http://guide.orthogate.com/workshops/email/orthlist.html.**

Bulletin Boards

A bulletin board is a space on a Web site where anyone can post a message and start a thread of discussion. When the next person visits the board, he can read and reply to that message. This is open to anyone who is given the address of the site. The messages are not sent out to anyone but remain on the site. The existing bulletin boards on some of the professional association sites are not widely used. The Orthogate site has been re-configured to a news/bulletin board format (**http://www.orthogate.com**).

Discussion Groups

Although the orthopaedic community on the Internet seems to use e-mail lists more than anything else for discussion purposes, there are other options. A discussion group is a Web site that is dedicated to a specific topic, such as the sports medicine site on the American Academy of Orthopaedic Surgeons site. In many cases these sites are limited to members of the association. For a short period there was a Newsgroup (sci.med.orthopedics) but it folded because the need to moderate the contributions was too heavy a burden. The American Academy of Orthopaedic Surgeons maintains member-only discussion groups on their Web site. Go to **http://www.aaos.org/wordhtml/discuss.htm** The topics are:

Alternative/Complementary Medicine
Board of Councilors
Foot and Ankle
Hand
Hip and Knee
Infections
Orthopaedic Rehabilitation
Organizational Issues in the Practice of Orthopaedic Surgery
Pediatrics
Shoulder and Elbow
Spine
Sports Medicine
State Orthopaedic Societies
Trauma
Virtual Reality for Orthopaedic Surgeons

Antivirus Software

One of the most distressing problems is to have a virus invade your system through your e-mail program. There is a wide range of viruses, from a very benign virus that is more of a nuisance, to an extremely virulent variety that may wipe out your hard drive. I have had a virus that resulted in the loss of all my laptop data, including some wonderful pictures taken at the pyramids at Chichen Itza in Mexico. This is one of the downsides of digital photography; there are no negatives to reprint the lost pictures. Back up your data as soon as possible.

There are two main software programs for antivirus protection, Norton antivirus at **http://www.symantec.com** and McAfee at **http://www. mcafee.com.** Both of these companies offer software that you can install on your computer. The original program can be purchased in most computer stores or purchased online and downloaded if you are connected to the Internet. You then must keep the program updated with regular upgrades to prevent the latest and nastiest virus. The option that I prefer is to use the online version of McAfee that updates my program daily at 1 AM. My DSL line is continuous-on and the program updates each day. On several occasions I have had a virus that the installed software did not pick up, but was only found by remotely scanning my computer online from the McAfee site. This is a very inexpensive service, $29 per year, that more than pays for itself with continuous and current protection. Online virus protection is available at **www.mcafee.com.**

If you are using a continuously on Internet connection such as the DSL phone line or cable, you need to install a firewall to prevent malicious attack on your computer system by a hacker. I use a router with a firewall. This distributes my high-speed line to the other home computers, and protects the system against an invasion through the open line. I also have a wireless network set up, so that I can roam around the house with the laptop using the same high-speed connection from my main desktop computer.

PDAs—Personal Digital Assistants

If you thought that these little handheld devices were just fancy address books, you are behind the times. Now when I synch my Palm each morning, I get not only my up-to-date address book, but also all my activities for the day, and the latest news from CNN, *The New York Times*, and *PC World*. This is updated each morning through Avantgo (**www.avantgo. com**), a free Web-based information service.

So, what is available in the handheld market? Table 5.1 lists the comparisons of the four top-selling models, which are shown in Figure 5.12. The Palm was one of the first, 16 million devices sold, and one of the most popular PDAs (personal digital assistants) (Newton by Apple was in fact the first, but was discontinued by a poor marketing decision). With only a monochrome screen, low storage, and poor delivery, the Palm had serious competition from the Visor. Now there are several other devices to rival the Palm. This technology is going to have the greatest growth in the next few years by converging with the cell phone. The Samsung 1300, the Handspring Treo, and the Kyocera QCP 6035 are all examples of a "smartphone" that combine the Palm OS and a wireless phone. The newer devices with more storage and better screens have left the Palm a little behind. The Visor, one of the main competitors, is a little cheaper, but about twice the size, and uses the Palm operating system. The new Visor has more peripherals and uses the smart media storage card. Pictures can be taken on an Olympus camera, and viewed in a slide show on the Visor. The Visor can also be used to control your PowerPoint presentations on the laptop with a USB connection. Margi (**www.presenter-to-go.com**) has taken that one step further and you can present directly from the palm to the LCD projector. The new Sony device, CLIE PEG-N710C, is really a good multimedia PDA using the Palm OS with a memory stick for storage of pictures, music, and video. The other competitors are the IPAC by Compaq, the Jornada by HP, and the Casio, which all use the Pocket PC operating system from Microsoft. This is a scaled-down mobile version of the main Microsoft products: Outlook, Word, Excel, Reader, Internet Explorer, and WINDOWS™ Media Player. There is going to be a real battle in the next few years to see which of the operating systems wins the majority of the market share, Palm or Microsoft.

Several of the mobile phones, Samsung, Kyocera, and Handspring, have the Palm operating system and the phone integrated as one device. It is going to be the most interesting to see how this technology convergence plays out. The advantages of these devices are that they come on instantly to give you quick wireless access to the Internet for e-mail, Avantgo (a Web-based information center), and the Palm applications such as address book, notes, to-do lists, calendar, databases, and Epocrates (a drug information database).

What is the easiest way to get started? Go to the site **www.pdamd.com**, shown in Figure 5.13, and order the medical edition with all the appropriate software loaded.

So, what applications are available on the PDA? The most important function is to have immediate access to the phone and address book. Currently you have to open the PDA, find the number, and dial it on the phone. This is where convergence with the cell phone is going have the greatest benefit. The to-do list and memo pad are very handy to use with the pen-like device (stylus) to write the notes on the screen. There are programs that actually store the written scribbles or notes in the same style that you used. Most of the time the graffiti function is used to write on the screen. If you have to record any amount of data, then purchase the fold-up keyboard. I use this to enter databases and to write longer documents. A program called documents to go (**www.dataviz.com**) can translate a Word document into the Palm OS. The documents are compressed, without for-

TABLE 5.1. Comparison of the four popular PDA models.

PDA model	Palm 505	Sony 760C	IPAC 3850	HP Jornada
Size	Palm is the smallest, easily fits in a pocket	Slightly larger than the Palm	Largest, no longer fits in a pocket with the expansion sleeve	Palm sized
Battery	Rechargeable Longest battery life	Rechargeable	Rechargeable Shortest battery life	Removable rechargeable
Screen	Only marginal screen brightness Write on screen in graffiti or actual writing with add on program	Brightest and best screen resolution for pictures 320×320 Screen is larger than Palm Write on screen in graffiti or actual writing	Has biggest screen with good brightness by backlight from both sides Write on screen by tapping on keyboard or actual script Screen writing can be combined with dictation of short notes	Bright screen, backlit on only one side, slightly smaller than compact Has same screen function to type or write
Operating system	Palm OS 33 Mb 8 Mb memory	Palm OS 33 Mb 64 Mb memory	Pocket pc 64 Mb memory	Pocket pc 64 Mb memory
Programs	Address book Date book Expense Mail Memo Note pad To-do list All synch with Windows Outlook Palm reader Photosuite (still images and video)	Address book Date book Expense Mail Memo Note pad To-do list All synch with Windows Outlook Gmovie—video program Audioplayer PG pocket for still images	Address book Date book To-do list Outlook mail Windows media player (for audio and video—with external speaker) Internet Explorer Notes Excel Word PowerPoint player	Same programs as Compaq

	Avantgo, Epocrates, Documents to go (synch word and excel files)	Conflicts with some programs	Book reader, Easily synchs with Microsoft office programs including Outlook	Targus keyboard
Keyboard	Portable full-sized keyboard available	Portable full-sized keyboard available	Targus portable keyboard can be attached	
Expansion card	Multimedia is the secure digital card—64 Mb	Memory stick up to 128 Mb	Multimedia is the secure digital card—64 Mb. Expansion sleeve available that holds cards up to 5 gig	Built-in slot for flash memory cards up to 5 gig
Multimedia	Plays video slowly from expansion cards. No audio	Plays quick time compressed video from the memory stick. Easy to load on computer and transfer to PDA. Audio needs earphones, no external speakers	Plays video and audio, at acceptable resolution. Can fill the screen with image. Microphone allows dictation to notes and listening to video clips. PocketTV plays mgeg video	Plays video and audio, at acceptable resolution. Can fill the screen with image. Microphone allows dictation to notes and listening to video clips. Pocket TV plays mgeg video
Connection	USB. Wireless. Infrared transfer between Palm OS	USB. Wireless. Infrared transfer between Palm OS	USB. Wireless with bluetooth. Can infrared to Palm OS	USB. Infrared. Wireless with bluetooth
Ease of use for beginner	Good, but difficult to add the 3rd party programs to make it function like the pocket pc	Same as palm. Easy to add mp3 and video files with Sony software. Works well with Sony computers and cameras that use the memory stick	Easy to set up and configure if you use Windows and Outlook as your mail server	Easy to set up and configure if you use Windows and Outlook as your mail server
Cost	$400 US approx	$500 US approx	$600 US approx	$600

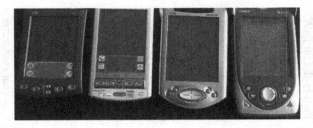

FIGURE 5.12. The four common PDAs: Palm 505, Sony 760, IPAC 3850, and HP Jornada 560

matting, to a very small file, about 10 to 20 Kbs. It is loaded on the PDA the next time you synch. You can use a portable keyboard and work at about the same speed on the Palm keyboard using only the PDA. This means that you only have to carry around two small devices instead of the laptop. If you are taking notes at a meeting, the PDA and the keyboard are much faster, smaller, and lighter than the laptop computer. At meetings the small size is not as distracting and noisy as a laptop.

The drawback in the past has been the small storage size on the Palm,

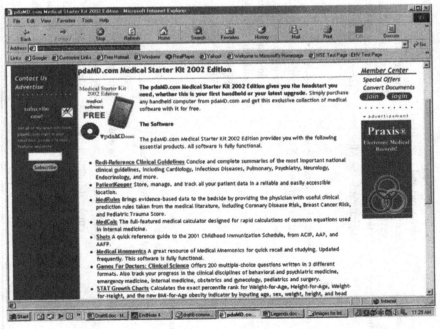

FIGURE 5.13. The pdamd site that sells the Palm preloaded with medical software

only 8 Mb. The new Palm 505 has expansion cards that increase the storage to 64 Mb. Now images and short videos may be stored on the card and shown on the Palm screen. The Visor, Sony, and Compaq devices all do the same with plenty of memory storage for images and video. The expansion cards are also available for Bluetooth wireless connections.

The other valuable feature for physicians (only available on the Palm OS) is the Epocrates drug information program. This program has every drug listed with dosages and interaction with other drugs, and is updated weekly. Now a vast pharmacopoeia is in your Palm with instant access to dangerous drug interactions. Most of the medical students, interns, and residents find this the most useful software (**www.epocrates.com**).

The orthopaedic residency program at Winston-Salem uses a PDA to synch the patient lists every morning for rounds. I have seen a program that will work with an Internet-based program called slimresidency (**www.slimresidency.com**) to provide a surgical log book, on-call scheduling, and other house staff chores. The PDA synchs this information every morning for the surgical house staff.

A similar function can be set up on the AvantGo Web site (**www. avantgo.com**). A folder of information may be created with daily news

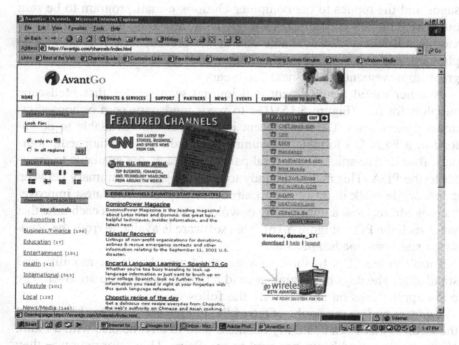

FIGURE 5.14. The AvantGo channels that can be downloaded to the PDA

and events that you can synch to each day as shown in Figure 5.14. This may be expanded to news, weather, stock market, and other nonmedical uses. The real advantage to this Internet-based program is that once it is configured, nothing more need be done. The PDA sits in the cradle, connected to the computer, which is on and connected to the Internet; the synch button is pushed, you get a coffee, and all the information for the day is loaded. This applies to the house staff, who need their assignments, and to the staff who need to know the meetings of the day and perhaps the news of the day.

The HanDbase (**www.ddhsoftware.com**) database programs for the Palm OS are very easy to use surgical databases. Up to 30 fields may be created to store information on surgical patients. These databases are instantly accessible and searchable for any of the data fields that you require. I keep about a dozen different databases such as interesting cases for rounds, PCL cases, and a complete surgical database. At the present time, 511 patient records only take up 81 Kb of space on the PDA. These databases are printable from the computer.

The PDA can download all your new unread e-mail messages in the morning and you can read them on the screen and reply to them as required. The next time that you synch, the PDA will transfer the new messages and the replies to the computer Outlook e-mail program to be sent out. The Palm OS does support a modem on the Palm 7 version. This service is not universally available and at the present time it is slow. The phone-based e-mail is also slow, but in both these areas I would expect great improvements in the next few years.

Another useful development is a journal scan service that Medscape supplies for free (Figure 5.15). Go to **www.medscape.com** orthopaedics, under journal scan. The most recent journal scans are available to download in a Palm OS format. The summaries of the main orthopaedic journals, four or five articles of several paragraphs each, are available to transfer to the PDA. This makes it handy to read the journal summary between cases, while stuck in traffic, in an airport or airplane. The latest improvement is Mdirect that automatically downloads the summaries each time that you synch the PDA (Figure 5.16). This software is available from the Medscape site **www.medscape.com**.

I look to the PDA to show us what the future holds for mobility and small size. The days of lugging around a nine-pound laptop are over. The main applications on the PDA are the following.

Address and phone book. One of the unique features that I like about the Palm is that I can beam my business card to anyone else with a Palm, Visor, or Sony and beam her card to my Palm. This information is then

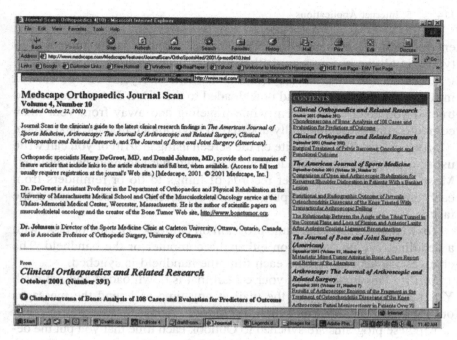

FIGURE 5.15. Medscape journal scans

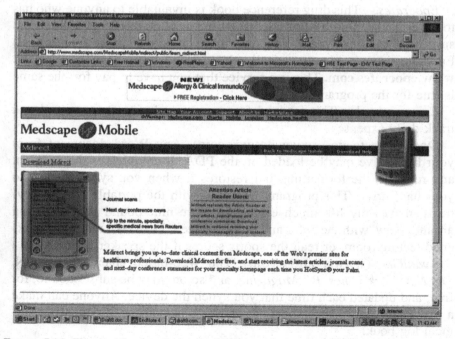

FIGURE 5.16. The download page for the Mdirect software to transfer the journal scans automatically to your handheld

entered into my address book. This makes it much easier compared to typing in all the business cards that I get at each meeting.

Calendar. All the daily events for the next five years can be entered into the Outlook program and downloaded to the PDA. The reverse is also true: if you enter a new event while traveling and away from your main computer, this is automatically updated to the computer on the next synch.

Memo pad. You can write on the screen using graffiti or you can write using a program that records your very own hard-to-read handwriting! Most of the memos are brief records of things to do or reminders from each day. These are easily purged from the system as you complete the tasks.

To-do list. This is the same program on Outlook. The major task, with a deadline, can be entered on either the computer or the handheld. The changes are kept up to date each time the handheld is synched.

Mail. This loads any of your e-mail that is downloaded and not read. You can read and reply to the mail at any time and send the messages out the next time that you synch the PDA.

All these programs are synched to Outlook each time that you put the device in the cradle and push the hot synch button. The newer devices connect through the USB port rather than the serial port, which is a bit slower.

Epocrates. This drug reference book is invaluable to anyone who has to order medications. (After you have been a sports medicine orthopaedic surgeon for a few years, you only have to know about four drugs!) Epocrates is updated automatically about once a week from the Web site **www.epocrates.com.** This is a service that you have to pay for; the same is true for the program.

Expense book. This is good for someone who needs to record and track daily expenses.

Documents to go (**www.dataviz.com**). Any Word document from your hard drive may be loaded on the PDA. It compresses the program and removes the formatting, but restores it when you synch it back to your hard drive. This program combined with the portable folding keyboard makes my life much easier, no more nine-pound laptops to lug around. Now, with the color and lighted screen, I can take notes in a darkened lecture room, or read the sports scores if the speaker is boring!

AvantGo (**www.avantgo.com**). The Web-based channels of CNN, *The New York Times, PC Magazine,* and so on, may be subscribed to, for free, and updated each time that you synch the device. Anyone can make a new channel for his personal use and keep a database of patients or surgical log book.

HanDBase. This is another one of the 1000 or so programs designed for the PDA. The vast number of Palm programs makes this the most appealing operating system. HanDBase (**www.ddhsoftware.com**) is a database that allows you to enter up to 30 fields. It is useful for a surgical log book, to keep track of interesting patients, or to make a list of patients for rounds. The residents can keep their surgical log book on this PDA-based database.

Access database.   A compression program is available to allow you to transfer your access database to the Palm. This takes quite a bit of space and is a good use for the expansion cards.

To access more medical programs for the Palm go to **www.pdaMD.com.**

Patient Care—What Is The Future?

In the future, the PDA may become more than just a reference tool for drugs and databases. It could well be the answer to prevent drug prescription errors. The transfer rate of data has improved with wireless technology. The prescription can be transferred from the Palm by infrared directly to the nursing station computer or via the modem to the pharmacy, either real or virtual. This system is far more reliable than the present handwritten paper prescription. There are still too many errors in interpretation of physician's handwriting that can be disastrous.

Physicians are slow to embrace any digital technology, as evidenced by the very few using electronic medical records in their offices. Industry has suggested that 20% of the younger generation of in-training physicians are using PDAs. The future lies with these physicians, but it may have to be legislated by the government to ensure compliance. This is similar to the notice that all physicians received several years ago in the Canadian system, that stated only electronic billing will be accepted; if you don't use the computer, the account will not be paid. The insurance companies who are paying out large amounts for medication errors may even demand it. Medication errors were the second most common payment claim over the past seven years. If you want to lower your risk, use electronic prescribing. There are several companies marketing handheld prescribing systems: Allscripts (**www.allscripts.com**), DocPlanet.com (**www.docPlanet.com**), ePhysician (**www.ephysician.com**), iScribe (**www.iscribe.com**), and Autros Healthcare solutions (**www.autros.com**).

Frequently Asked Questions About PDAs

1. *Question:* I currently keep multiple scraps of paper with notes on them of things to do. Is a PDA better or just more expensive? In what way?

Answer: The PDA is a more convenient and accurate way to jot down all the little memos that you collect during the day. In that way you have all those little scraps in one place. For years I used a Daytimer and wrote everything down with a pen. Once I switched to the electronic version, I wondered how I ever functioned without it. The messages may be downloaded to your computer to expand or to save.

2. *Question:* Is a PDA easy to leave lying around?

   Answer: Yes, you can lose the PDA. I have left one in a rental car and had it returned. I have been using the Palm for five years and only lost it once, on an airplane. I keep it in my pocket, one of the reasons that I favor using the smaller Palm version compared to the Visor. If you synch regularly with your desktop, you won't lose much critical information. If your PDA is password-protected, privacy is not compromised even if you lose it.

3. *Question:* Is dealing with e-mail on the PDA really a good idea? Will the synch work for all e-mail programs or only Outlook?

   Answer: E-mail is still a function that I prefer on the computer. I can get confused enough using several computers and multiple e-mail addresses. In the future the convergence with a high-speed phone connection may make this more appealing.

4. *Question:* What is the advantage of an updatable calendar if I have to have my secretary type up the events?

   Answer: This is the one function that I like the most about the PDA. I have the next five years of activities all recorded on my Palm and can immediately check what I am doing next week or next year. I think that this is an important-enough function that I do it myself on the desktop and synch it to the Palm daily.

5. *Question:* It is a legal requirement to protect patient privacy. What precautions must be taken to make sure your PDA cannot "leak"? How much of a problem is this?

   Answer: I use a patient database on the Palm to record all my surgical cases. I have the Palm protected with a password to prevent this information from being distributed.

6. *Question:* How does prescribing by a PDA work? There are issues of connection and compatibility. Is there a system at the pharmacy end that will receive my prescription in electronic form?

   Answer: At the present time this is one of the potential future uses for the PDA. This may never become a reality for many of the reasons that are suggested. However, we should consider how what we do now can be improved with an electronic version, similar to the electronic operative report that incorporates the digital images and video.

7. *Question:* There seems to be a clash of operating systems between the Palm OS and Pocket PC. Which side will win? Should I wait until the convergence of PDA and cell phone has got a bit further?

Answer: This is a reasonable worry. The best PDA by Apple, the Newton, was discontinued before it really had a chance to compete. The Palm OS is the most widely used at the present time and will probably survive in some form. The future is the convergence with the cell phone, but this is an even bigger question as to who will control the market. You just have to jump in and get your feet wet and at $150 for a bottom-of-the-line Palm to do your notes and calendar it hardly matters.

8. *Question:* If most of the purpose of a PDA is to do with text, what is the point of a more expensive color screen?

Answer: I used the Palm V for several years and only switched to the Palm 505 this past year. The difference is like day and night (forgive the comparison). The screen can now be seen in marginal situations, like a lecture hall with the lights down, in an airplane, taxi, and so on. I now can take notes in a lecture theater with the portable keyboard and have replaced my laptop. Just like the Palm device itself, once you have used a color-lighted screen, you won't go back. The latest Palm version also shows video. So now you can show a video clip of a pivot shift test to the students in the clinic before they exam the patient. I can visualize that in the future you would be able to download a video clip of the surgical procedure that you are about to perform.

In the future, PDA use will be similar to the current use for the laptop.

Becoming a Presence on the Web

What Is a Web Site?

A Web site is a collection of linked .html pages. The first page is the home page to introduce the site. Navigation buttons are usually listed down one side to describe what the site is about, who runs the site, what services are offered, and, for commercial sites, what product is for sale, how to order the product, and how to contact the company. The strength of the Web site is the linking of many pages together. Usually words that are colored and underlined are linked. Thus, **www.aana.org** will link you from this page to the Arthroscopy site. By using the back button on the browser, you can return to previously visited pages. You can also locate the site by bookmarking a page in the browser and returning at any time to the same page.

A Web site is also an opportunity for you as a practitioner to make yourself known and interact with patients and potential patients. The ISOST Guide has a valuable discussion of the reasons for setting up your own practice Web site (**http://guide.orthogate.com/chapter4.html**). This may vary from person to person and from one nation to another. In general, even surgeons who have little need to recruit patients to their practice could use a Web site to reduce the burden on their patients and themselves with information about orthopaedic conditions and "frequently asked questions" FAQ pages. In the USA there is more emphasis on promoting one's practice but a mix of patient information is offered too. There is great concern about the poor quality of "orthopaedic information" on the Internet. Practice Web sites help with this problem both by providing good information and by directing patients to other sites of which you approve. The patient information sites presented in Appendix 1 and on the OWL Patient Information Page offer an enormous variety of sites with expert and highly reputable provenance. If you can make a simple Web page, you can direct your patients to Internet resources that you personally have approved.

How to Make Web Pages

The easiest way to make Web pages from a word-processing document such as MS Word is to "save as" a Web page in your word processor. The easiest way to edit a Web page is to purchase a program such as FrontPage from Microsoft. This looks just like any word-processor page. You type the information on the page, in a format called WYSIWYG (what you see is what you get). As we saw in Chapter 1, native HTML can get to look complex. FrontPage is much easier for the novice to learn.

It used to be that the Internet was the realm of the nerds, who would later grow up to be computer programmers. You had to take a course in "How to Write in HTML." That was a little like learning DOS. In the early days, I went to several courses to learn both DOS and HTML. Now, of course, FrontPage looks just like MS Word. If you know how to use a word processor, you can write HTML pages. In other words, writing Web pages is really a secretarial function. An extensive workshop on creating Web pages is posted at **http://guide.orthogate.com/workshops/webedit/default.htm.**

The more complex aspect of designing Web pages is how to add images, link topics and pages together, and post these on a server. I still maintain my own Web site and add information and new pages through a process called file transfer protocol (FTP). This is a process of transferring files from one computer to another over the Internet. This basic process of writing HTML on FrontPage is very simple, and I leave the more complicated server management issues to a professional company.

Instead of designing your own Web pages, you can hire a company. The cost of setting up a basic Web site will vary from $1000 to $5000 depending upon the complexity of the site. If you want to do any secure online business transactions or maintain a database, this is going to be more expensive.

If you want a basic orthopaedic site, you can obtain one for free if you are a member of the American Academy of Orthopaedic Surgeons. They have a service on their Web site that allows you to enter information on templated HTML pages that are then assigned a URL. For instance, both authors have a site on the Academy Web site: **http://orthodoc.aaos.org/ DonJohnsonMD/** and **http://orthodoc.aaos.org/MylesClough/.** The addresses signify that we have Web sites hosted on the **www.aaos.org** server. We can then link to all the Academy patient information. This address can be given to our patients and we can be assured that they will get high-quality orthopaedic information approved by the Academy. The basic problem with these "off the shelf" Web sites is that they only offer patient information that the parent organization provides. The surfing tradition of the Internet means that most patients want to derive information from a number of sources. One page on a topic doesn't cut it. It would be better, but much more difficult, to offer patients a wide variety of approved information sites so that they come back to your site again and again to find the links and don't go off to the search engines to swim with the sharks before they have obtained a solid grounding.

Most physicians do not have the time or the expertise to create and manange their own Web sites. There are several providers that will set your office up with a Web site to provide a variety of levels of services and patient information. They usually have a considerable amount of patient information that can be linked to your pages. Your patient is given the URL and can access the information that you control. A good example of this service is Active Life Network at **www.activelifenetwork.com**. I have set up a Web site with them called **www.anteriorcruciateligament.com** allowing me to link to their ACL information. Several of the orthopaedic equipment companies will also supply information related to their areas of expertise. For example, Linvatec (**www.linvatec.com**), an arthroscopy equipment manufacturer, has partnered with WebPartners to host **www.aclsolutions.com, www.shouldersolutions.com,** and **www. kneesolutions.com**. These sites can provide your patient with information about the anterior cruciate ligament. So you see, there is really no excuse for not having a Web site of your own. You may not need it, but the patients need and expect you to have a Web site address. The process of setting up a Web site varies from the basic inexpensive information about your office or clinic to a major multimedia extravaganza. It all depends on how much you want to spend or how aggressively you want to advertise. I have had someone tell me that 75% of his cash-only orthopaedic referrals comes from his Web site! Now, that's marketing.

These are a couple of examples of private orthopaedic Web sites that have become successful:

www.scoi.com—Southern California Orthopedic Institute, and
www.stoneclinic.com—the home page of Dr. Kevin Stone.

Digital Imaging

If you are going to get involved in the Web site business, you need to acquire digital images to put up on your site. Maybe it is something as simple as a picture of your clinic, a map of directions on how to get to the clinic, or a picture of the attending staff. So how do you get a digital image? The process consists of three parts: acquisition, editing, and archiving of images. A workshop on capturing, editing, and using orthopaedic digital images is at **http://guide.orthogate.com/workshops/imaging/default.htm.**

First of all what is a digital image? In a digital image all the information about the colors and shapes is encoded as numbers not as tiny dots of color on a film or piece of paper. Although you can convert a normal photograph into a digital image by scanning it, you can also acquire a digital image immediately by digital photography. This is the process of acquiring an image without the use of traditional film. In the film process, light is exposed to a film embedded with hundreds of millions of silver halide crystals. The film is developed with chemicals and indicates how much light was exposed on the film. The negative is used to expose the same amount of light on a photographic paper that is then developed to create an image as seen through the camera lens. A digital image is acquired by focusing the image on a rectangular array of tiny light and color sensors. Each sensor records the information for one pixel of the image, so the more pixels, the better the quality of the image.

Can digital photography be as good as film? Digital and traditional are complementary arts, and both have their advantages. Digital is ideal for instant gratification, and that fits with most orthopaedic surgeons' personalities. A slide has 12 million color dots which are equivalent to pixels of information. The best digital cameras now have a 6-million pixel CCD.

A 4-million pixel image can produce an 8 × 10 print that is indistinguishable from a print of the same size. So digital is close to slide resolution for most of the uses that we have at present. For presentation on a computer screen there is no difference between digital and traditional photographs. There are usually only 800 × 600 pixels (480,000) on a computer screen. So your high-quality photograph is 25 times too detailed to be seen on one screen and your medium-quality digital image is 8 times too large. Both will have to be resized with consequent loss of image information to be viewed on a computer screen.

What Are the Main Uses of Digital Photography?

The main use in orthopaedics is to document the patient's current status. In arthroscopy, a digital image is taken before and after surgery. The clinical photo of the patient's knee is done before and after surgery, for example, before and after high tibial osteotomy. The degree of hyperextension can be documented. The X-rays before and after surgery can be recorded. This information may be stored in a patient file to be accessed at any time in the future. A slide show of the images can be done for the patient, and a PowerPoint presentation of the images can be made for rounds. A printout of the images can be given to the patient or stored in the patient's chart. The digital images can be embedded in an electronic (HTML page) operative report such as Notematic from **www.puremed.com** and stored on the Internet. Medical/legal reports with images included are worth much more to the lawyers.

How Do You Acquire a Digital Image?

Digital images can be made from traditional film cameras by scanning the slide or photo into a software program such as PhotoShop on the computer. Flatbed scanners may be used for photos and slide scanners for slides. If you have a lot of slides, it is easier to take them to a Kodak photo shop and have them scanned to a CD. This will cost about a dollar a slide, but it eliminates the time-consuming process of hand scanning each of the slides. Scan in only the high-quality clinical or X-ray photos. Any of the text slides can be redone in PowerPoint much more efficiently.

A digital camera is the other easy method to acquire digital images. Most of the high-resolution cameras cost about $800 to $1200. This will give you two to three megapixels, a zoom lens, macro capability, and storage on a digital flash memory card. The capture card is removed and a card reader is used via a USB port on the desktop or through a pcmcia reader for the laptop. The card shows up as a removable drive when the "my computer" is opened. The removable drive is opened and the images dragged and dropped into a folder on the hard drive. The subject of image acquisition is dealt with at **http://guide.orthogate.com/workshops/ imaging/capture.htm.**

Photo Editing

Once the photo has been scanned in, or transferred by memory card from the camera, it should be imported into a photo editing program such as PhotoShop, PhotoDeluxe from **www.adobe.com,** LightView pro from **www.lview.com,** or PhotoImpact from **www.ulead.com.** The image may be lightened, darkened, cropped, rotated, given a file name, and stored as a JPEG, BMP, TIFF or in several other image formats.

Common Editing Tasks.

- Conversion of color to grayscale (monochrome). This is only necessary for X-rays but is a very good thing to do with them. It eliminates the greenish tinge from the fluorescent screen. It also reduces the size of the file substantially.
- Cropping. On a normal X-ray and in most clinical pictures there is a lot of space on the image that conveys nothing. If storage space or the cost of sending files over the Internet is an issue, you don't need the parts of the image that don't convey any useful information. Crop them out.
- Rotation. Bones look better straight up and down. With an image editor you can nearly always rotate the image until the appearance is pleasing.
- Brightness. We often use a bright light to view X-rays. Many times a digital image will be too bright or too dark when you view it on the monitor. Image editing programs all allow you to adjust the brightness and the (trickier) contrast. Make sure you know how to undo a change because you can spoil the image.
- Color manipulation. If you have taken a clinical photograph in fluorescent light, a more natural color can be obtained by adjusting the color curves or the hue. It takes some practice to do this and it is different from one image editor to another. PhotoDeluxe has an option in the image quality menu called Instant Fix which does quite a good job.
- File conversion. No matter what format the image was loaded as, the program will usually allow you to store it in a different format. You choose when you "save as" and are choosing a file name. Make sure to select the file format at the same time (Figure 5.17).

Note that you can select the format you use to store the image. Some of these formats are compressed, saving space but potentially losing image quality. Others are uncompressed and take up a lot more space.

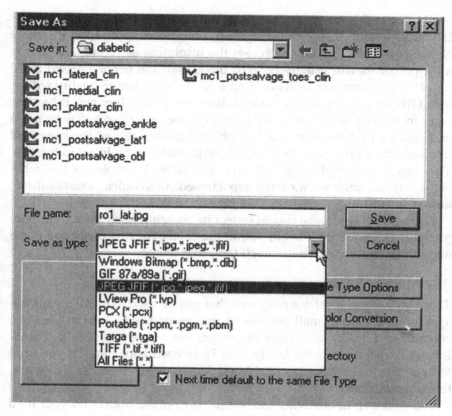

FIGURE 5.17. Lview image storage dialog box

We have talked a lot about space and file size in this section on image editing. This is because it is considered bad manners to send overly large images over the Internet. A big image cannot be seen on one screen so the recipients of your images will have to edit them to see them. In some parts of the world ISPs charge by the kilobyte for information transmitted. So people pay 50 times more for a 1-Mb image they cannot see without manipulation than they would for a 20-Kb image with all the same information. The Digital Image editing overview is at **http://guide.orthogate. com/workshops/imaging/edoverview.htm,** and a detailed workshop is at **http://guide.orthogate.com/workshops/imaging/editing.htm.**

A further word about file formats. If you are going to print an image, save it as a .BMP or .TIFF file. This is a larger uncompressed file, but prints well. The resolution should be set at least 200 to 300 dpi to print. Now this is going to be a large file and should only be done if you may need to print this image, for example, for publication in a journal article. If you are going to use the image in a computer application the other choice is to compress the image, set the resolution at 72 dpi, and save it as a jpeg. This will usually be 1/10 the size of the uncompressed BMP file. If you convert the JPEG back to a BMP, some image quality will be lost. GIF format is used for colored diagrams on the Internet. It has one other interesting application, GIF animation. Several photos may be taken in sequence of a dynamic exam, such as a drawer test of the knee, and inserted into a program that cycles these pictures much like a video clip. This makes a normally static photo come alive. Examples of this technique may be seen at **www.carletonsportsmed.com/clinical_examination_ animations.html**.

The name of the image should reflect its contents, such as "acl-chronic-partial-tear.jpg." Then I could search the folder for that name and come up with several images with much the same theme.

Archiving the Images

There are several database programs that can be used to archive your images. If you have a small number of images and only need to view the contents of a folder to retrieve an image, use a program such as Photo-Impact Explorer as shown in Figure 5.18 (**www.ulead.com**). If you need to search a large database of 20,000 images, use Thumbsplus (**www. thumbsplus.com**).

The first step in archiving the images is to make folders on your hard drive. Have a copy of these folders on your server or backup disc to make retrieval easy. The arthroscopy knee images, for example, are stored under subfolders of ACL, PCL, Meniscus, Chondral, Patellofemoral, and so on.

Once you have a lot of images in the folder you need to be able to search the folder for the image that you took last year of the chronic ACL tear. WINDOWS XP™, WINDOWS™ 2000, and WINDOWS™ ME come with a function to view the contents of the folder as thumbnails. This will allow you to access the folder quickly, but if the number of pictures becomes large this can be tedious. There are several programs that will display thumbnails inside a folder. PhotoExplore from **www. ulead.com** will also allow you to delete, rotate, and do some image correction to each of the photos in the folder. You can make a slide show of all or some of the images. Light view Pro from **www.lview.com** will also display thumbnails and do a slide show of the contents of the folder. Image Access Pro was the best program to search a database, but is no longer supported by **www.scansoft.com.** This was an access database and could

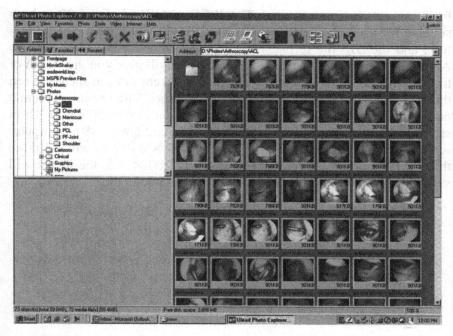

FIGURE 5.18. View of the thumbnails of the arthroscopy images in the Arthroscopy/ACL folder on the hard drive

catalog thumbnails, do a slide show, and allow you to search by keywords or by title of the image. An excellent searchable database can be created with Thumbsplus available from **www.thumbsplus.com**. This is the program that is currently recommended.

Uses of Digital Imaging

The electronic record of the patient's condition before and after treatment is essential. In arthroscopy most of the procedures are done without any permanent record. The status of the joint before and after surgical treatment should be documented. This can be stored as hardcopy from the printed images in the patient's record, or stored on a server in digital format. The digital video that has been captured at the same time may also be stored with the patient's file. The before and after digital X-rays may also make up part of the record. These may be stored in a folder that is archived by Thumbsplus, Image Access pro, or by Photo Explore.

The images may be used to make a rounds presentation in PowerPoint. This same slide may be used later for an academic paper presentation on the same subject. The images also may be incorporated into a Web page for a presentation on a subject. The JPEG or GIF file formats are both suitable for the Internet. The compressed JPEG is best for a clinical picture, and the GIF file format for a colored drawing. Programs such as Adobe Image Ready (included in PhotoShop) will give you the length of time it will take to download the image at different modem speeds. Keep this in mind when posting images on the Internet. The resolution should be low, 72 dpi, and the image size can be kept low at 50 to100 Kb in size. Most images can be smaller than the standard 640 × 480. Computer screens generally run at 1024 × 768. The 640 × 480 size will fill more than half the screen. If you cut this down to 300 × 225, the image will still be usable, but will have a much faster download time.

6
Orthopaedic Web Pages

Introduction
Prime Sites—Orthopaedic Surfboard

Introduction

The task of selecting orthopaedic sites to include in a list of this sort (Appendix 1) is daunting, humiliating, and ultimately futile. It is daunting because the Orthopaedic Internet has grown far beyond the size where any one or even any organization can keep track of it. Despite five years of constant effort a review of the OWL collection of links reveals a humiliatingly incomplete account of what is available. There are many subjects not covered in this list. It's not because they are not covered somewhere on the Internet. It is because a mechanism for keeping up with the growth of the Internet has not yet matured. The printed list is also futile because anyone planning actually to use the list will want the URL addresses in a form that the browser can use as links. No one expects readers to copy out hundreds of Web addresses. The CD-ROM has this information in link form and should be used for any exploration of the Orthopaedic Internet. Even the CD-ROM has a frustrating element to it. Without maintenance, any static list of links will become rapidly obsolete as the Internet changes. Between August 2001 when OWL was last updated and October 2001 when this was written, at least 10% of the links were lost. If you believe that this list is of value you will find that the posted version (Orthopaedic Web Links, OWL) grows as people send in sites of interest and is, at least intermittently, updated.

This collection, then, is a personal snapshot of the 2001 Orthopaedic Internet to offer you some understanding of the depth and variety of the material known to the authors. It is a certainty that the reality is deeper by far and enormously more various.

Prime Sites—Orthopaedic Surfboard

The sites in this section represent, in the authors' opinion, the most informative, interesting, and innovative sites on the Orthopaedic Internet. If you have doubts about the value of the information available on the Internet or believe that everything on the Net is rubbish, we recommend that you surf through these sites before deciding there are no valuable resources. All sites can be accessed without cost although some do require registration.

Wheeless' Textbook of Orthopaedics

You may never get past this site! C.R.Wheeless' revision notes were tidied up and posted as a set of interlinked Web pages (Figure 6.1). The coverage of topics from Head Injury to Mallet Toe is extremely thorough. In the five years since this site was first posted more illustrations have been added, as well as guest pages and outlinks to many other resources. The only valid criticism that has been leveled at this site is that it was written by a resident. This is only partly true as Wheeless probably drew

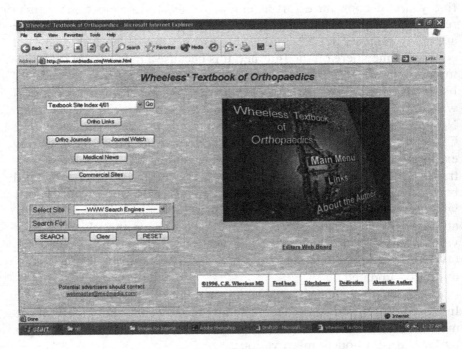

FIGURE 6.1. *Wheeless' Textbook of Orthopaedics*

much of his material from handouts prepared by the teaching staff at Duke. Almost all the great orthopaedic textbooks started as the notes of a resident and it is tempting to predict that this one will keep up the tradition.

WorldOrtho—The Ultimate Orthopaedic and Sports Medicine Web Site

The "Educational Database" of WorldOrtho (Figure 6.2) contains several textbooks on orthopaedics, trauma, and sports medicine. It also contains "Core Topics in Orthopaedics," lecture notes, several quiz sites, and a photographic tour of the "examination of the musculoskeletal system."

The Comprehensive Classification of Fractures of Long Bones

Posted by AO North America (Figure 6.3), this site makes the "AO classification of long bone fractures" easy to understand and use as a reference. Each bone is divided into segments, usually proximal, diaphyseal, and distal. For each segment the fracture types are further explained with

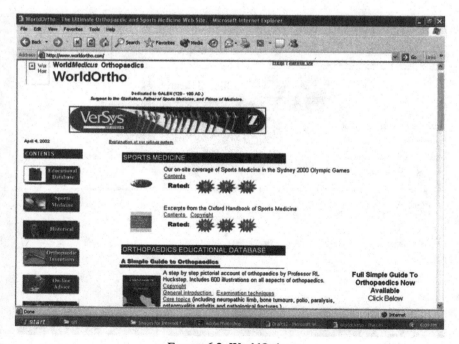

FIGURE 6.2. WorldOrtho

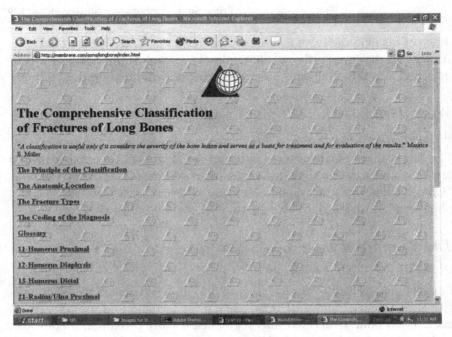

FIGURE 6.3. AO Classification of fractures of long bones

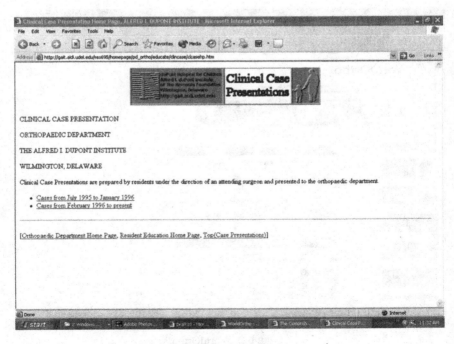

FIGURE 6.4. DuPont Institute case presentations

A being simple fractures and *B* and *C* being multifragmentary fractures. The site goes on to describe the classification for each long bone region.

Clinical Case Presentations. DuPont Institute

These case presentations (Figure 6.4) were made by residents in the DuPont Hospital training program. They cover a wide variety of pediatric orthopaedic topics, presenting a well-illustrated case, offering a didactic account of the condition, and a review of the literature. They are fine examples of what every teaching program should be doing on the Internet. This kind of scholarship is presented every day in different programs; unless it is posted it is lost.

Carleton University Sports Medicine Clinic

This site, shown in Figure 6.5, offers a wide variety of educational resources for physicians and patient information pages with the focus on sports medicine and especially knee reconstruction. There is a useful collection of arthroscopic images from the author's extensive collection. This is one of the pioneer sites on the orthopaedic Internet.

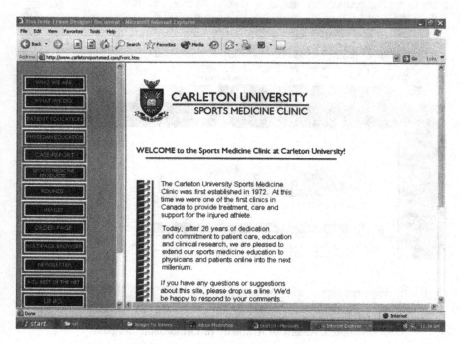

FIGURE 6.5. Carleton University Sports Medicine Clinic

American Academy of Orthopaedic Surgeons

The AAOS site (Figure 6.6) is surely the leading institutional site in orthopaedics. It has a huge amount of information accessed from a cleverly crafted home page that has direct links to nearly 100 other parts of the site without the appearance of clutter. Highlights of the site include the patient information section, information about the annual meeting (including past and present abstracts), and the full text presentation of the *Bulletin of the AAOS*. "Find a surgeon" gives the office addresses and Web sites of AAOS members in every nation, US state, and Canadian province. The members section has full text access to the AAOS journal and to a site that will prepare and post a practice Web site for each member. Recently added is "Orthopaedic Knowledge Online" (OKO), which consists of a selection of topics treated in depth. Currently the selection is small and the material seems to be derived from articles from the *Journal of the AAOS*. This site, which has enormous potential, is accessible to all fellows and international affiliates of the AAOS.

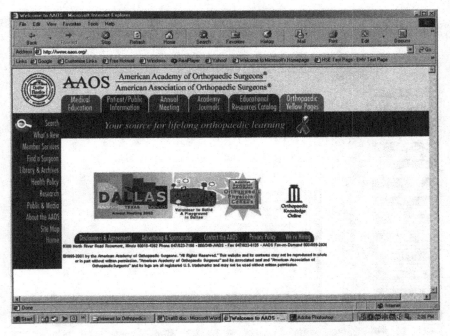

FIGURE 6.6. American Academy of Orthopaedic Surgeons

Belgian Orthoweb

This pioneer site (Figure 6.7) is edited by Jan Van Der Bauwhede and Dick Vandelvelde. When it started in 1996 it was the first site to try to bring the Orthopaedic Internet activities of most of the professional societies of one nation onto the same site. Now the journal *Acta Belgica Orthopaedica*, the Orthopaedic Association, the Arthroscopy Association, the Arthopaedic Trauma Association, the Hand Group, the Pediatric Orthopaedic Association and the Foot Surgery Society are all hosted on the same site. The BeneluxOrth Mailing list is also hosted and there is an extensive collection of case presentations. The European mirrors of *Wheeless' Textbook* and Orthogate are hosted there also. The editors have been active and influential in the Orthogate project.

e-Hand

This enormous site (see Figure 6.8 for its contents page) provides a fantastic resource for hand surgery. Edited by Charles Eaton, the site offers a solid account of the subject. As an example, the hand surgery gallery

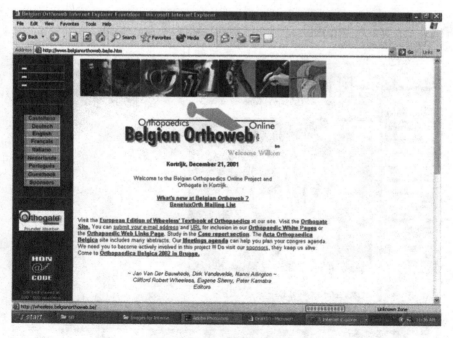

FIGURE 6.7. Belgian Orthoweb

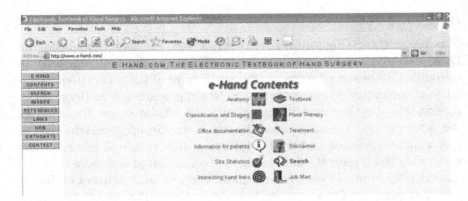

FIGURE 6.8. e-Hand table of contents

has over 2000 images of cases. The classification home page is particularly useful. Dr. Eaton has been an active member of ISOST and moderates the hand surgery e-mail list. He has provided many of the "Cases of the Week" problem cases sent to the list.

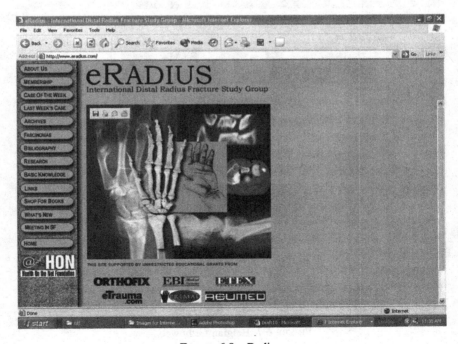

FIGURE 6.9. eRadius

Distal Radius Fractures eRadius

This is perhaps the most specialized site on the Orthopaedic Internet, a large, well-organized site entirely devoted to one condition—distal radius fractures (Figure 6.9). Cases are presented and critiqued by world-famous authorities on the subject. Access requires (free) registration.

Medscape Orthopaedics Home Page

For orthopaedic surgeons wishing to keep up with current issues in orthopaedics, Medscape offers articles written by experts in the field, often reviewing the presentations at recent meetings (Figure 6.10). Medscape is a commercial site paid for by advertising, but access to the information is free once you have registered. The contents page does not give access to all the orthopaedic articles. You can use the site's search engine or browse under the headings of News, Clinical Updates, Surgical Management, Resource Centers, Medscape Mobile (PDA programs), Practice Guidelines, Medical Image Center, Conference Coverage, Course Reports, Conference Schedules, CME Center, Journal Room, Exam Room,

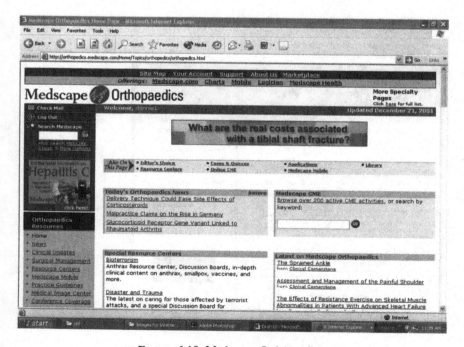

FIGURE 6.10. Medscape Orthopaedics

Grand Rounds, Multimedia Library, Patient Resources, and Managed Care. Some of the pages offer CME credit.

The Orthopaedist's Guide to the Internet

This site was prepared by the Internet Society of Orthopaedic Surgery and Trauma (ISOST) to offer basic and advanced information about the Internet to orthopaedic surgeons (Figure 6.11). The sections include information on the use of e-mail, imaging, searching the Internet, setting up an office Web site, finding orthopaedic suppliers' Web pages, orthopaedic discussion forums, and Web page editing. The tutorials on these subjects are freely available online, and the examples and problems described are ones familiar to orthopaedic surgeons.

OWL, Orthopaedic Web Links

OWL (Figure 6.12) is the largest collection of links to subjects of interest to orthopaedic surgeons on the Net. Originally formed by the amalgamation of three major collections maintained by orthopaedic surgeons,

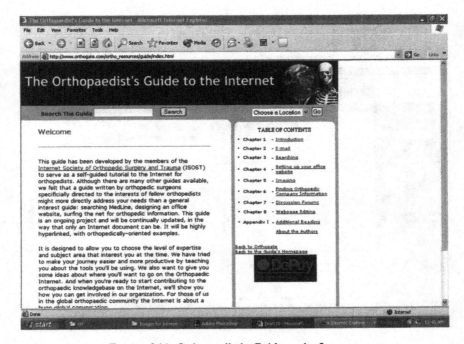

FIGURE 6.11. Orthopaedist's Guide to the Internet

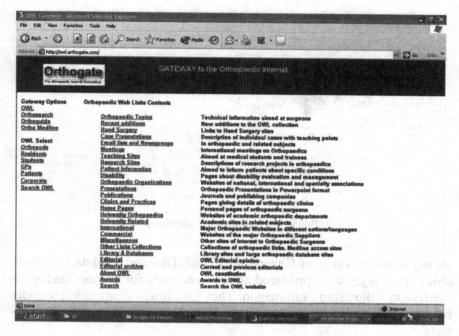

FIGURE 6.12. Orthopaedic Web Links (OWL)

it now forms the center of the Orthogate Project, an attempt to provide an academic and practical core to the Orthopaedic Internet. The OWL collection has two guiding principles: the link is "straight-to-the-meat" whenever possible, avoiding navigation from the front page; and all indexed pages have been selected by an orthopaedic surgeon. "OWL Patient Information" pages, for example, are selected from the information provided by organizations such as the AAOS, American Academy of Family Physicians, university sites, and orthopaedic surgeons' Web sites. Thus it offers variety, with information from many resources, and security that the origins are reputable and professional. Of more direct interest to orthopaedic surgeons are the "Orthopaedic Topics" pages that link directly to sites on the Internet aimed at informing and educating orthopaedic surgeons.

South Australian Orthopaedic Registrars' Notebook

These notes (Figure 6.13) were produced by orthopaedic trainees at Flinders Medical Centre in South Australia. They cover 55 different top-

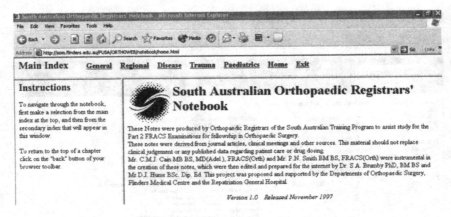

FIGURE 6.13. Registrars' Notebook

ics under the headings of General, Regional, Disease, Trauma, and Pediatrics. The pages were produced as revision notes for trainees taking the Australian Fellowship examination. They lack illustrations and references but form an interesting counterpoint to Wheeless' entries on the same subjects.

Orthoteers

The Orthoteers site (Figure 6.14) is also a collection of revision notes suited to the requirements of candidates for the Irish FRCS examination. It covers this syllabus in sections entitled Clinical Examination (e.g., a whole page on the Trendelenburg test, how to perform it, and what to expect in different conditions), Pediatric Orthopaedics, Foot and Ankle, Hand and Wrist, Elbow, Humerus, Shoulder, Basic Sciences, Spine, Hip and Pelvis, Knee, Orthopaedic Infections and Microbiology, Rehabilitation, Orthopaedic Pathology, Perioperative Issues, Trauma, and Extras. The site is password-controlled but registration is free. The overall quality of the information is good, with some illustrations and relevant links to other sites on the Internet.

ORCID Orthopaedic Rare Conditions Internet Database

Each orthopaedic surgeon sees a number of rare conditions every year; the problem is that they are never the same rare conditions! We tend to cope with the problem by reading up about the subject and using that expertise to treat the patient to the best of our ability. Since we never see another case, this expertise is soon dissipated. ORCID (Figure 6.15) was

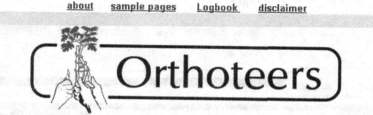

about   sample pages   Logbook   disclaimer

Welcome to **the Orthoteers Orthopaedic Education Resource** - The largest Orthopaedic e-textbook on the Web.

This site was developed for Postgraduate Orthopaedic Trainees preparing for the FRCS (Tr&Orth) Examination in the United Kingdom. It is also open to others after joining and getting password access.

If you would like to access the site, please **complete the Membership Form**. For an example of the pages in the site **Follow this Link**

The Trainees Surgical Logbook is available for **Download HERE**.

Please enter your password:

Submit

If you do not have a Password you can join here:

Membership Form

FIGURE 6.14. Orthoteers

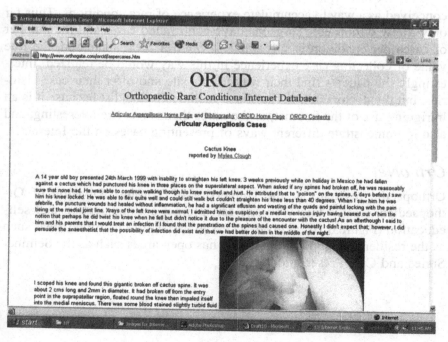

FIGURE 6.15. Cactus spine in the knee: a case from ORCID

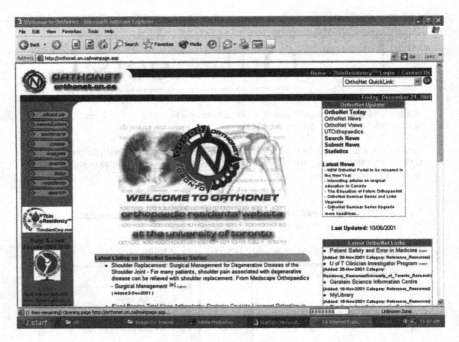

FIGURE 6.16. Orthonet

conceived as a way to accumulate experience of rare conditions. Thus far only a few orthopaedic surgeons have contributed cases and the number of cases per condition is still small. If both of these increased, the true value of collecting case experience in this way would be realized. Interestingly the patients find their way to this site and offer their case histories, but the doctors don't. The site is included in this list because it is an intriguing use of the Internet, as the cases themselves are interesting, and also to demonstrate different ways of presenting cases on the Internet.

OrthoNet

Orthopaedic residents at the University of Toronto, Division of Orthopaedics, created this Web site for internal communication and self-education (Figure 6.16). It gives access to password-controlled areas such as the residents' logbooks, but it also has open areas such as the Seminar Series and Case Presentations.

7
The Future of the Orthopaedic Internet

Introduction
A View from the Future
    Personal Changes
    Relations with Patients
    Feedback and Communication
    Research Communication
    Orthopaedic Teaching
    Redundant Effort
Clearinghouse for Orthopaedic Information

Introduction

Although the Internet has not yet assumed a dominant role in orthopaedic communication and academics, the speed with which things are moving in that direction makes it likely that it will. A change comparable to that which occurred after the introduction of printing is upon us. It's doubtful if Gutenberg's fellow burghers could have sat down and predicted the Renaissance, the Reformation, the growth of science, and the flowering of literature. How could they have foreseen religious wars, propaganda, pornography, and cultural extinction? But if they could and had taken a few insightful actions, just think how much trouble might have been saved! Business as usual when a tidal wave of change is approaching is simply nonsensical. Now that the Internet has demonstrated its potential and some of its problems, we need to consider the changes that are likely to occur in our subject and how we should react.

A View from the Future

There is a technique in physics for solving difficult theoretical problems. One assumes the answer is correct and searches for the phenomena that would exist if it were. From a study of those phenomena one may often gain insight into the process and finally make the proof by a backdoor approach. We are going to apply a similar approach by assuming the future and then think about how to get there from here.

If technological civilization survives, we are assuming that a computer network will be the dominant provider of information in the twenty-second century. When faced with a need to obtain more information on an orthopaedic subject, the first step would be to interact with a site to define exactly the subject in which you are interested. This would take you to a level of granularity that might be exemplified by "predictors of outcomes after different forms of treatment for a Pipkin I fracture dislocation of the femoral head." The network would have a classification system that would consult with you to establish exactly what it is that you wished to research. Once you have mutually established that, the system would ask whether you wish a consensus view, whether you want to know the issues and controversies surrounding the topic, or whether you want up-to-date research data about it. The output options would thus be a limited number of sites offering the current consensus, a larger number of sites covering the issues, a connection to the main research thread on the subject, or, finally, access to all the information around on the subject arranged into "folders" as Northern Light does.

The information then made available to you would be a layered presentation with a simple summary on top from which you could explore down to the bedrock of data if you so wished. Competing and contrasting points of view would be offered and unresolved controversies identified. There would be no doubt where "evidence-based practice" was and where controversial treatment options began. In addition, case presentations and the addresses of experts on the subject who were willing to give advice could be found by the same search process.

Now, what are the structural components that would have to exist for such a system to work and be valuable? The least obvious of these is a universally accepted classification of orthopaedic subjects. English is a rich language with many ways of saying the same thing; and it is only one of hundreds of major languages. If you are looking for avascular necrosis, you must recognize that aseptic necrosis, osteonecrosis, and AVN plus all the terms in other languages must be brought into the search paradigm. The simplest way to achieve the precision needed to start a comprehensive search is to generate a code. The dialogue between searcher and the system can take place in any language and go via any route but it would end up with a unique code for every orthopaedic topic. Then the system uses the code as a search string. In our glimpsed future we assume that anyone who posts information and who wants people to find it will know that they have to include the subject code in the title or keywords of the document. They will also know that notification of the search site is a critical step once they have posted the new document. The search site will look for the code not the words. Both from the point of view of those searching for orthopaedic information and those posting it, there should be only one gateway site. Everyone who wants to find orthopaedic information and everyone who is offering orthopaedic information will be literally "on the same page."

The second less-than-obvious conclusion is that achieving this is a people problem, not a technical problem. The computer techniques to achieve all this exist already and are being put to daily use in many of the sites we have discussed. Although advances in artificial intelligence might make a difference, the main problems are the economic, institutional, and organizational barriers. We need people to review sites and to determine "best practice" and the consensus; we need editors of research threads and moderators of discussion groups; we need people who will organize research projects over the Internet. And these people must be orthopaedic surgeons with experience in teaching and leading our subject; we are not going to accept the opinions of librarians, generalists, or self-appointed dot-com entrepreneurs. The greatest challenge is to create an academic body with information technology expertise, whose orthopaedic opinions will be respected.

The authors of this book are among the small group of orthopaedic surgeons who predicted that this would occur sooner or later and have been working to ensure that it is "sooner" and that the development is controlled for the benefit of orthopaedic surgery and our patients. A gateway site that would more or less control what people found out about orthopaedic surgery on the Internet is one which could very easily be misused or abused. The work of keeping up such a site is well beyond what an individual could accomplish, and an individual gatekeeper makes no sense anyway. So the next corollary of this view of the future is that an organization of orthopaedic surgeons must come together to create, maintain, and guard the gateway. Until this organization becomes stronger than the tiny group of "orthogeeks" who meet annually during the AAOS meeting, development will be stalled.

Personal Changes

We have known for some time that it is impossible to keep current with more than a small corner of orthopaedics; yet our patients expect that we are current in whatever problem they face. To a large extent the information is out there on the Net but if it's not in our heads we either ignore it, or feel ashamed that we have to go look. Both options are dangerous. Now that looking things up is easy and rapid, we should recognize that it is more appropriate than relying on memory. This has implications in personal habits, education, and CME. Far from creating information overload, the Internet offers a solution, an ectopic brain. We have to change our behavior to accommodate that. Perhaps for 90% or even more of our cases what we "know" is enough and we don't have to rush to references to treat every hip fracture. Yet, even with hip fractures there are still surprises, else why would we still be doing research on the subject. Another personal change we may need is a reminder to review common problems once in a while, or some form of "push" technology to prod us when a significant change in the knowledge base arises.

Another valuable change would be recognition that we are members of a global community and that there are friendly, helpful people out there who would be pleased to offer insight into the problems you share with your patients. The orthopaedic e-mail lists have been described as the "Global Corridor Consult," and this description does give the flavor of the interaction.

Relations with Patients

This is the biggest part of the tidal wave. We are going to have to relate to patients who have researched their own personal problem in great detail. Their confusion may be greater than their understanding but they will be much more persistent than we are over seeking out everything they can find. Trying to ignore that or urging them to ignore this source of information will not work for long. Instead we will need to look for productive ways to form partnerships with inquisitive patients and make them into research assistants. As a first step, we should guide them to reputable resources. But we should accept and encourage further exploration, as long as they discuss what they find with the treating team. We need to be frank in recognizing that they may find out some things new to us in this process. This may be a big change for surgeons. The prevailing attitude is still "I'm the doctor; I know what is best for you." A more appropriate stance might be, "I have expertise on your problem; it's my job to give you the information you need to make the treatment decision which is right for you."

With that attitude the Internet is a reality check: does what I say to my patients gibe with what they find on reputable sites? But there's no denying that it is more work. Nor that I am poorly prepared for a patient pointing out something I didn't know. I know that I don't know things but do I want my patient to know that? But we cannot put the genie back in the bottle. We are committed to dealing with inquiring patients who will make more work for us; we must make sure we and they get value for that work. We might consider saying to a patient, "You have such severe arthritis of the hip that the only thing which will make much difference is an operation. Here is a list of sites with information for people in your position. Come back in a week and we will discuss it further; I will answer any questions to the best of my knowledge and will pursue any open questions. E-mail me if you run into any problems as you go along. You are the person who decides what to do based on our joint learning and my advice." That is the relationship we foresee as becoming common and indeed being desirable.

There are a couple of corollaries. The first is that we must be active in ensuring that good information sites are out there and that orthopods in general know where they are and can/will direct their patients there. Which brings up the questions of, "What is good?," "Who says so?," and "How do I find them?" We should expect organized orthopaedics to establish what should be covered on a patient information site; another expectation is getting patients themselves involved in the evaluation of sites. These are all issues that require a clearinghouse for orthopaedic information on the Internet.

The second corollary is that restricting patients to approved sites won't work; if they want to, they will swim with the sharks. So shark recognition kits should be issued and survivors' narratives heeded. The AAOS is doing a significant service by providing good-quality patient information and more organizations need to do the same. It will never completely satisfy the patient's thirst for information, though. If I develop osteolysis of my hip replacement, I am not going to be content with what the AAOS tells me—or my doctor, or Dr. Huddlestone, or the Rothman Institute, or Zimmer. I will want to make my own synthesis and see if my doctor agrees.

Feedback and Communication

Feedback is so easy on the Internet but the attitudes that inhibit it remain. "Who-am-I-to-have-an-opinion?" is very prevalent and has earned the few of us who are less inhibited about offering advice a rapid and no doubt undeserved reputation as gurus. This ought to change. When a colleague asks you a question in the corridor you give an answer. The Internet allows the sum of those answers to add up to something quite a lot more valuable. We are not saying we should be flooded with "I agree" messages but we need the behavior change that permits us to offer thoughtful opinion without being inhibited.

Research Communication

Who knows how this is going to develop? The journals offer priceless experience and editorial and review skills, but little of that is paid for. Instead we pay through the nose for what we don't need: printing and distribution. Commitment to the "paper" model also prevents us from pursuing several innovations made possible by IT. One is the concept of a layered presentation instead of a sequential one. We do this already by skimming the methods unless we dislike the results and feel the need to discredit the findings. In a hypertext presentation the top layer could be a summary couched in terms that a lay person could understand but which would convey to the expert what the research is about and what the new findings are. Lay people are going to read abstracts anyway so we may as well take advantage of that. The next "layer" would be much more like our current Introduction/Methods/Results/Discussion format but split up into small chunks so that if people want to refer to your work they can link directly to the point they want to cite rather than make the reader go through the whole thing. At an even deeper layer you might expect the database that was analyzed to produce the conclusions reported. Thus if someone wanted to redo the statistics or do a meta-analysis it would be easier.

The second innovation would be open peer review. We all accept that peer review is valuable and necessary but it takes place in secret. In part this is to reduce the humiliation of authors and in part it is to protect the anonymity of reviewers. We should loosen up a little and accept that the editing and reviewing function is a way to improve the work. If we bring the process into the open, we can see the comments of the editors and reviewers and most importantly add our own. In this way the work will really be reviewed by peers, not just by a secret coterie. Instant feedback and easy updating allow us to do this. It would still be the responsibility of the editor finally to accept or reject the piece of work and incorporate it into the "journal," but we would all learn more from an open process. *Editorial Peer Review: Its Strengths and Weaknesses* is the subject of a recent book by A.C. Weller (see a review in Medscape). She reaffirms the value of peer review but points out significant and disturbing unanswered questions such as, "Is there an exact, measurable benefit of editorial peer review? Do researchers from major institutions and departments publish more because of a bias in their favor or because they produce a better piece of research or scholarly communication?"

The third innovation would be the concept of research as a thread. At the moment we do the work, write the paper, accept the editor's and reviewers' amendments, and do the proofs; at last it is published and we draw a line underneath (at least in our own minds). But it shouldn't be like that. A good piece of work should set up numerous new questions and provoke a stimulating discussion that would lead to new work or an expansion of the old. If all the researchers who are interested in the same subject contributed to the same ongoing discussion, how much easier it would be for the rest of us, trying to form an opinion that helps us take care of patients. This is so self-evidently valuable, it is achievable with current technology, so the pressure to build these institutions will be irresistible. Journals and journal editors should be experimenting with new formats and ways of presenting orthopaedic research information; many of them are. The Nature Publishing Group maintains an interesting forum on electronic publishing with many diverse points of view represented. The flashpoint at the moment is the issue of copyright. The publishing houses insist on the retention of copyright as a commercial asset to maintain the viability of the journals. Those in favor of free transfer of information argue that the copyright should revert to the authors after a period of time to allow free posting of the information.

Orthopaedic Teaching

The orthopaedic trainee acquires a knowledge set concerning orthopaedic conditions and their treatment; a skill set, to do with surgical technique and patient evaluation; and a mind set, to do with how to manage orthopaedic problems and the person to whom they are attached. The knowledge set is changing rapidly, and the mind set we currently teach is not well adapted to the IT world. Even the skill set changes, but not as fast. We need to teach trainees to rely on their memory less than on looking things up, to know how to find the information they need, to join in discussions when they have a worthwhile opinion, and to see research as a thread and information as a seam to be mined. (*The Information Age: Implications for Orthopaedic Education*, Christian Veillette, MD, and Edward Harvey, MD. Canadian Orthopaedic Web site at **http://www. coa-aco.org.**) We need to make sure they enter into an information partnership with their patients, where they do the leading but expect surprises from their followers.

Redundant Effort

Every day around the world many minor and some major efforts of scholarship are being wasted. The reading list, the presentation at rounds, the seminar, even the medico-legal opinion require that someone with significant orthopaedic knowledge and skills sets about reviewing a subject and "writing it up" in some form or other. Then the message is delivered and may make an impact on the audience but goes no further. Turning that piece of scholarship into a paper or a chapter in a textbook is such an enormous effort that it is very rarely done. Yet it is easy to post on the

Internet and examples such as *Wheeless' Textbook* and the Dupont Institute series of "Rounds Presentations" show how valuable such collections of minor scholarship can become. Then the next person who needs to review that subject can get a flying start and devote his energies to improving the work rather than starting from scratch.

Implicit in this process of iterative improvement of reviews of orthopaedic subjects is the concept of a clearinghouse for information so that someone who want to use and improve the treatment of the topic can find the current "best" version. Yet another needed behavior change is that people who post or update orthopaedic information should notify the clearinghouse. That goes for people who make valuable literature searches or Internet searches. There is no need to have to repeat them.

Clearinghouse for Orthopaedic Information

The need for such an institution is clear but it is much less clear how it will rise to a position of authority. We need one site where users can go with a reasonable expectation of being able to find what they are looking for and reasonable certainty that it will be on subject and of acceptable provenance. That same site would be the natural place for providers of orthopaedic information to notify about their postings. Mechanisms of comment, bibliographies, iterative reviews, research threads, and many of the other helpful innovations can develop around a clearinghouse. Without one it's difficult to see how they can.

A clearinghouse for orthopaedic information will be much more than a list of links. Because of the traffic expected it would be valuable commercially, but because it would need to act for the benefit of orthopaedic surgeons and ultimately of their patients, it would need to have solid academic and institutional backing. To put it another way, we need agreement from the national and international orthopaedic organizations that a clearinghouse is necessary and serves the interests of their members. Because the Internet is international, even the most powerful national body cannot accomplish this task on its own.

The Internet Society of Orthopaedic Surgery and Trauma (ISOST) was founded in 1999 to promote the development of an orthopaedic clearinghouse and to educate orthopaedic surgeons in the use of information technology. It is a nonprofit society with bylaws modeled on the Hip and Knee Society. The officers are barred from profiting by the activities of the society. Using its Orthogate site, the society has fostered the embryos of the institutions that may grow into a viable clearinghouse. These include the Orthopaedic Web Links (OWL) collection of links to orthopaedic subjects on the Internet, the Orthopaedists' Guide to the Internet with teaching files and workshops, and the Orthogate Patient Information collection which serves as a yardstick. There are orthopaedic special interest mailing lists hosted on the site with archives and an image bank. OCOSH, the Orthogate Classification of Orthopaedic Subject Headings, is also posted as we believe that the accurate classification of subjects and images on the Internet will be a necessity if we are to find them. Perhaps ISOST's most valuable role is to show what can be done. It is far from certain that the orthopaedic clearinghouse envisaged in our view from the future will actually grow from this effort.

Other ways would include the commercial route. There are already dozens of commercial sites that would like to be the "one gateway" to medicine on the Internet. The attractiveness of the commercial prize makes it unlikely that any one site will become dominant enough to act as a clearinghouse and it seems unlikely that orthopaedic surgeons would willingly give that sort of power to a commercial organization. Another alternative would be for a major national organization such as the AAOS to devote resources to providing a clearinghouse for American orthopaedics. Because of the number of users in the USA this might become a dominant institution and other nations would have to "join in" once it became clear that following their own path would not serve their members as well. Lastly we suppose that the effort could be international in origin from the beginning with SICOT providing the impetus. On ideological grounds one might hope or prefer that competing institutions might vie with each other to set up the best possible service. There is certainly value in choice. However, keeping up with new postings on the Internet is inherently impossible unless the gateway site is notified. That is only likely to occur if one site predominates.

Meanwhile ISOST will continue to provide an example and may grow. Perhaps one of the most necessary changes in the behavior of orthopaedic surgeons would be to pay attention to these issues and make sure that they are not settled by default. The Internet doesn't need to be promoted by orthopaedic surgeons; it is self-evidently valuable. But orthopaedic surgery on the Internet does need promotion and fostering to make sure that it grows and develops in ways best adapted to our subject and our challenging times.

Appendices

Appendix 1
Orthopaedic Internet Resources
Appendix 2
Health-Related Internet Resources
Appendix 3
Departments of Orthopaedic Surgery: Domestic and International

Appendix 1
Orthopaedic Internet Resources

1. *Wheeless' Textbook of Orthopaedics*. You may never get past this site! C.R.Wheeless' revision notes were tidied up and posted as a set of interlinked Web pages. The coverage of topics from head injury to mallet toe is extremely thorough. In the five years since this site was first posted more illustrations have been added, as well as guest pages and outlinks to many other resources. The only valid criticism that has been leveled at this site is that it was written by a resident. This is only partly true as Wheeless probably drew much of his material from handouts prepared by the teaching staff at Duke. Almost all the great orthopaedic textbooks started as the notes of a resident, and it is tempting to predict that this one will keep up the tradition.
http://www.medmedia.com

2. *WorldOrtho—The Ultimate Orthopaedic and Sports Medicine Web Site*. The *Educational Database* of WorldOrtho contains several textbooks on orthopaedics, trauma, and sports medicine. It also contains *Core Topics in Orthopaedics*, lecture notes, several quiz sites, and a photographic tour of the examination of the musculoskeletal system.
http://www.worldortho.com

3. *The Comprehensive Classification of Fractures of Long Bones*. This is posted by AO North America. This site makes the AO classification of long bone fractures easy to refer to and understand. Each bone is divided into segments, usually proximal, diaphyseal, and distal. For each segment the fracture types are further explained with As being simple fractures and Bs and Cs being multifragmentary fractures. The site goes on to describe the classification for each long bone region.
http://membrane.com/aona/longbone/index.html

4. *Clinical Case Presentations. DuPont Institute*. These case presentations were made by residents in the DuPont Hospital training program. They cover a wide variety of pediatric orthopaedic topics, presenting a well-illustrated case, and offering a didactic account of the condition and a review of the literature. They are fine examples of what every teaching program should be doing on the Internet. This

kind of scholarship is presented every day in different programs; unless it is posted it is lost.
http://gait.aidi.udel.edu/res695/homepage/pd_ortho/educate/clincase/clclasehp.htm

5. *Carleton University Sports Medicine Clinic*. This site offers a wide variety of educational resources for physicians and patient information pages with the focus on sports medicine and especially knee reconstruction. There is a useful collection of arthroscopic images from the author's extensive collection. This is one of the pioneer sites on the orthopaedic Internet.
http://www.carletonsportsmed.com

6. *American Academy of Orthopaedic Surgeons*. The AAOS site is surely the leading institutional site in orthopaedics. It has a huge amount of information accessed from a cleverly crafted homepage which has direct links to nearly 100 other parts of the site without the appearance of clutter. Highlights of the site include the patient information section, information about the annual meeting (including past and present abstracts), and the full text presentation of the *Bulletin of the AAOS*. *Find a Surgeon* gives the office addresses and Web sites of AAOS members in every nation, US state, and Canadian province. The members' section has full-text access to the *Journal of the AAOS* and to a site that will prepare and post a practice Web site for each member. Recently added is *Orthopaedic Knowledge Online* (OKO), which consists of a selection of topics treated in depth. Currently the selection is small and the material seems to be derived from articles from the *Journal of the AAOS*. This site, which has enormous potential, is accessible to all fellows and international affiliates of the AAOS.
http://www.aaos.org

7. *Belgian Orthoweb*. This pioneer site is edited by Jan Van Der Bauwhede and Dick Vandelvelde. When it started in 1996 it was the first site to try to bring the orthopaedic Internet activities of most of the professional societies of one nation onto the same site. Now the journal *Acta Belgica Orthopaedica*, the orthopaedic association, the arthroscopy association, the orthopaedic trauma association, the hand group, the paediatric orthodpaedic association, and the foot surgery society are all hosted on the same site. The BeneluxOrth mailing list is also hosted and there is an extensive collection of case presentations. The European mirrors of *Wheeless' Textbook* and *Orthogate* are hosted there as well. The editors have been active and influential in the Orthogate project.
http://www.belgianorthoweb.be

8. *e-Hand*. This enormous site provides a fantastic resource for hand surgery. Edited by Charles Eaton, the site offers a solid account of the subject. As an example, the *Hand Surgery Gallery* has over 2000 images of cases. The *Classification Home Page* is particularly useful. Dr. Eaton has been an active member of Internet Society of Orthopaedic Surgery and Trauma (ISOST) and moderates the hand surgery e-mail list. He has provided many of the *Cases of the Week* problem cases sent to the list.
http://www.e-hand.com

9. *Distal Radius Fractures*. eRadius This is perhaps the most specialized site on the orthopaedic Internet, a large well-organized site entirely devoted to one condition—distal radius fractures. Cases are presented and critiqued by world-famous authorities on the subject. Access requires (free) registration.
http://www.eradius.com

10. *Medscape Orthopaedics Home Page*. For orthopaedic surgeons wishing to keep up with current issues in orthopaedics, Medscape offers articles written by experts in the field, often reviewing the presentations at recent meetings. Medscape is a commercial site paid for by advertising, but access to the information is free once you have registered. The contents page does not give access to all the orthopaedic articles. You can use the site's search engine or browse under the headings of *News, Clinical Updates, Surgical Management, Resource Centers, Medscape Mobile* (PDA programs), *Practice Guidelines, Medical Image Center, Conference Coverage, Course Reports, Conference Schedules, CME Center, Journal Room, Exam Room, Grand Rounds, Multimedia Library, Patient Resources*, and *Managed Care*. Some of the pages offer CME credit.
http://orthopedics.medscape.com

11. *The Orthopaedist's Guide to the Internet*. This site was prepared by the ISOST to offer basic and advanced information about the Internet to orthopaedic surgeons. The sections include information on the use of e-mail, imaging, searching the Internet, setting up an office Web site, finding orthopaedic suppliers' Web pages, orthopaedic discussion forums, and Web page editing. The tutorials on these subjects are freely available online, and the examples and problems described are ones familiar to orthopaedic surgeons.
http://guide.orthogate.com

12. *OWL, Orthopaedic Web Links.* OWL is the largest collection of links to subjects of interest to orthopaedic surgeons on the Net. Originally formed by the amalgamation of three major collections maintained by orthopaedic surgeons, it now forms the center of the Orthogate Project, an attempt to provide an academic and practical core to the orthopaedic Internet. The OWL collection has two guiding principles: the link is "straight-to-the-meat" whenever possible, avoiding navigation from the front page; and all indexed pages have been selected by an orthopaedic surgeon. *OWL Patient Information* pages, for example, are selected from the information provided by organizations such as the AAOS, American Academy of Family Physicians, university sites, and orthopaedic surgeons' Web sites. Thus it offers variety, with information from many resources, and security that the origins are reputable and professional. Of more direct interest to orthopaedic surgeons are the *Orthopaedic Topics* pages that link directly to sites on the Internet aimed at informing and educating orthopaedic surgeons. There are 7000 pages of orthopaedic content.
    http://owl.orthogate.com

Case Presentations. These 303 sites offer individual case presentations.
    http://owl.orthogate.com/Case_Presentations/index.html
Commercial Sites. These consist of 199 sites of orthopaedic supply companies and other related commercial sites.
    http://owl.orthogate.com/Commercial/index.html
E-mail Lists. These 18 sites of orthopaedic mailing lists have information on joining the list and browsing the archives.
    http://owl.orthogate.com/Email_Lists/index.html
General Lists. These are 149 sites of general orthopaedic interest.
    http://owl.orthogate.com/General_Resources/index.html
International. These 64 sites list the international orthopaedic sites.
    http://owl.orthogate.com/International/index.html
Orthopaedic Organizations. These comprise 154 sites of the professional orthopaedic organizations.
    http://owl.orthogate.com/Organisations_and_Associations/
    index.html
Orthopaedic Topics. These 3974 sites cover the major orthopaedic topics including the following.
    http://owl.orthogate.com/Orthopaedic_Topics/index.html
    Children's Orthopaedics — 223 sites of orthopaedic treatment of conditions that affect children.
        http://owl.orthogate.com/Orthopaedic_Topics/Paediatric_
        Orthopaedics/index.html

Conditions — 101 sites of common Orthopaedic conditions
**http://owl.orthogate.com/Orthopaedic_Topics/Conditions/
index.html**

Orthopaedic Complications — 48 sites of complications of orthopaedic conditions and treatment.
**http://owl.orthogate.com/Orthopaedic_Topics/Orthopaedic_
Complications/index.html**

Regional Orthopaedics — 2327 sites organized by region of the body, such as the knee, hip, spine, and so on.
**http://owl.orthogate.com/Orthopaedic_Topics/Regional_
Orthopaedics/index.html**

Sports Medicine — 71 sites dealing with orthopaedic treatment relating to sports injuries.
**http://owl.orthogate.com/Orthopaedic_Topics/Sports_Medicine/
index.html**

Trauma — 349 sites concerned with the orthopaedic treatment of trauma, fractures, dislocations, and ligament injuries.
http://owl.orthogate.com/Orthopaedic_Topics/Trauma/index.html

Tumors — 245 sites of tumors of soft tissue and bone.
http://owl.orthogate.com/Orthopaedic_Topics/Tumours/index.html

Patient Information. This consists of 1414 sites whose primary purpose is to supply information suitable for patients and family.
http://owl.orthogate.com/Patient_Information/index.html

Practice Web sites. There are 111 sites of orthopaedic clinics, practices, and homepages of orthopaedic surgeons.
http://owl.orthogate.com/Surgeons_and_Clinics/index.html

PowerPoint Presentations. There are 64 sites with PowerPoint presentations of orthopaedic subjects.
http://owl.orthogate.com/Presentations/index.html

Publications. There are 108 sites of orthopaedic journals and scientific publications.
http://owl.orthogate.com/Publications/index.html

Teaching Sites. These 388 sites are aimed at the orthopaedic resident or medical student.
http://owl.orthogate.com/Teaching_Resources/index.html

University Sites. These are 179 sites of university departments of orthopaedics.
**http://owl.orthogate.com/Universities_and_Academic_Centres/
index.html**

13. *South Australian Orthopaedic Registrars' Notebook.* These notes were produced by orthopaedic trainees at Flinders Medical Centre in South Australia. They cover 55 different topics under the general headings

of *General*, *Regional*, *Disease*, *Trauma*, and *Paediatrics*. The pages were produced as revision notes for trainees taking the Australian Fellowship examination. They lack illustrations and references but form an interesting counterpoint to Wheeless' entries on the same subjects. **http://som.flinders.edu.au/FUSA/ORTHOWEB/notebook/home. html**

14. *Orthoteers*. The *Orthoteers* site is also a collection of revision notes suited to the requirements of candidates for the Irish FRCS examination. It covers this syllabus in sections entitled *Clinical Examination* (e.g., a whole page on the Trendelenburg test, how to perform it, and what to expect in different conditions), *Paediatric Orthopaedics*, *Foot and Ankle*, *Hand and Wrist*, *Elbow*, *Humerus*, *Shoulder*, *Basic Sciences*, *Spine*, *Hip and Pelvis*, *Knee*, *Orthopaedic Infections and Microbiology*, *Rehabilitation*, *Orthopaedic Pathology*, *Perioperative Issues*, *Trauma*, and *Extras*. The site is password-controlled but registration is free. The overall quality of the information is good with some illustrations and relevant links to other sites on the Internet. **http://www.orthoteers.co.uk/**

15. *ORCID Orthopaedic Rare Conditions Internet Database*. Each orthopaedic surgeon sees a number of rare conditions every year; the problem is that they are never the same rare conditions! We tend to cope with the problem by reading up on the subject and using that expertise to treat the patient to the best of our ability. Since we never see another case this expertise is soon dissipated. ORCID was conceived as a way to accumulate experience of rare conditions. Thus far only a few orthopaedic surgeons have contributed cases and the number of cases per condition is still small. If both of these increased, the true value of collecting case experience in this way would be realized. Interestingly, the patients find their way to this site and offer their case histories but the doctors don't. The site is included in this list because it is an interesting use of the Internet; the cases themselves are intriguing and it demonstrates different ways of presenting cases on the Internet. **http://www.orthogate.com/orcid/contents.htm**

16. *OrthoNet*. Orthopaedic residents at the University of Toronto, Division of Orthopaedics created this Web site for internal communication and self-education. It gives access to password-controlled areas such as the residents' logbooks but it also has open areas such as the *Seminar Series* and *Case Presentations*. **http://orthonet.on.ca**

Appendix 2
Health-Related Internet Resources

Disease-Specific Sites
    Surgery
    Hand Surgery
    Minimal Access Surgery
    Orthopaedic Surgery
General Medicine
    Medical Internet Guides
    Aging and Gerontology
    Alternative Medicine
    Associations and Societies
    Cancer
    Communicable Disease
    Computers and Health
    History and Reference
    Medical Internet Guides
    Medical News and Information
    Medical Publishers
    Pharmaceuticals and Products
    Physiology
    Practice Management
General Interest
    Fitness and Exercise
    Living and Lifestyle

Disease-Specific Sites

Surgery

Hand Surgery

American Association for Hand Surgery
Research awards, established to "foster creativity and innovation" in hand surgery, are available from the American Association for Hand Surgery

to residents, fellows, and therapists. An application form can be found on the Web site, but must be mailed in after completion. Nominations may also be made for the Vargas International Hand Therapist Award, named in honor of Dr. Miguel Vargas. A calendar of events and conference information is obtainable on this site.

http://www.handsurgery.org

American Society for Surgery of the Hand

This organization provides continuing medical education through meetings, seminars, online skills, self-assessment programs, and publications about the hand and upper extremity. A listing of international meetings on hand surgery is included, along with contact information for those meetings. Often the meetings have their own Web page and those are duly linked here. A book and a video library are cataloged online. The public information section contains a *Find-a-Doc* section that lists (by state and name) local area surgeons with a specific interest in surgery of the hand.

http://www.hand-surg.org

British Society for Surgery of the Hand

This Web site, which is currently "under construction," contains a history of the organization, demographics for hand diseases, and the number of surgeons needed to treat them. A description of common hand problems, such as Dupuytren's contracture, rheumatoid arthritis, and soft tissue injuries is available. Fellowships are listed, as are current meetings. A list of support groups and other links to online resources is available.

http://www.bssh.ac.uk/

e-Hand, Electronic Textbook of Hand Surgery

Handling over 27,000 hits per day, this is surely one of the busiest of the hand surgery Web sites. Visitors may view the anatomy of the hand in great detail through online images on this Web page. Although the taxonomy system used to navigate the site can be difficult to use, the resulting graphics files (referenced to Primal Pictures) are quite well made and instructional. The *Handbase* case of the week archives contains two years' worth of monthly cases with high-quality images of radiographs and good discussions.

http://www.eatonhand.com

Hand Transplant

Matthew Scott, recipient of the first hand transplant performed in the United States, takes center stage on this Web page. Having lost his dominant hand in 1985 to a fireworks explosion, he underwent the transplant in January, 1999. Intraoperative photographs are available as well as an impressive picture of Mr. Scott using his transplanted hand to throw out the first pitch before the Philadelphia Phillies opening game just three months after the surgery. Future possible recipients can learn more basic facts online and may seek additional information by e-mail.

http://www.handtransplant.com

International Hand Library

An official repository for documents of the International Federation of Societies for Surgery of the Hand, this Web page contains a calendar of events including contact information for each event. The vendor market-place section is a comprehensive list of the products and services of interest to hand surgeons. Members of the organization can gain access to additional exclusive areas of the Web site. Cases may be submitted for discussion in some sections.

http://www.handlibrary.org

Minimal Access Surgery

International Society for Computer Aided Surgery

The goal of the International Society for Computer Aided Surgery is to advance the utilization of computers and related technologies in the treatment of patients. Visitors to the Web page may view a listing of members along with their e-mail addresses. Those seeking membership can fill out an online application. A list of society activities, including the annual meeting, is included. Sections on statutes and counsel are also available.

http://www.iscas.org

Orthopaedic Surgery

American College of Sports Medicine

The American College of Sports Medicine (ACSM) Web page contains a media room with news releases, quotes, *In the News*, and history sections. The meeting and continuing education sections list the upcoming scientific meeting with highlights and a nice summary of each meeting. A member service center explains the benefits of becoming an ACSM member, describes each of the membership categories available, and allows application for new or renewal membership. Links to online journals, brochures, video and audio resources, and reference guides are available.

http://www.acsm.org

General Medicine

Medical Internet Guides

Aging and Gerontology

Geriatrics

Access to the journal *Geriatrics* is available at this site.
   http://www.geri.com/

Alternative Medicine

Alternative Medicine Home Page

The *Alternative Medicine Home Page* is a jump station for sources of information on unconventional, unorthodox, unproven or alternative, complementary, innovative, and integrative therapies. When visited around the first of the year, the site had not been updated since August, but still contained a group of useful and current links.
   http://www.pitt.edu/~cbw/altm.html

Chiropractic OnLine

Chiropractic OnLine is presented as a public service by the American Chiropractic Association and contains a long list of resources for consumers, health professionals, and others.
   http://www.amerchiro.org/

Associations and Societies

American Academy of Orthopaedic Surgeons

This site provides both member and public access to topics of interest to orthopaedists and patients with orthopaedic concerns. Included are directories of specialists, an orthopaedics yellow pages, and information about meetings. Links to other medical sites and MEDLINE are available.
   http://www.aaos.org

American Academy of Pediatrics

Topics and membership benefits for the members of the American Academy of Pediatrics.
   http://www.aap.org

American Association of Health Plans

This site is provided by a trade organization representing HMOs.
   http://www.aahp.org

American Cancer Society

This site offers local and national cancer news and the ability to search the site for specific content. It includes a media services section that is interesting and a useful source of information for those in the media.

http://www.cancer.org

American College of Emergency Physicians

Member services and information for members of the American College of Emergency Physicians.

http://www.cep.org/

American College of Physicians (ACP)

The American College of Physicians (ACP) provides selections from ACP journals, CME, medical computing, managed care information, classifieds, Web site reviews, a product catalog, and more.

http://www.acponline.org/

American Health Decisions

American Health Decisions is a confederation of state health programs that assists in developing education programs about health care and policy. The group promotes patients' rights in medical care, including the right to refuse or accept treatment. It also conducts research on health care policy issues.

http://www.ahd.org

American Medical Association

This is the Web site of the American Medical Association. It provides health and fitness info for resources on conditions and family health.

http://www.ama-assn.org

American Medical Informatics Association

This Web site is designed to help answer questions about AMIA, its services, and activities. At this Web site, you can find out about meetings and educational events, membership in AMIA, AMIA's structure and operations, publications, medical informatics and related issues, and background information about previous meetings.

http://amia2.amia.org/

American Medical Women's Association

This national organization supports the advancement of women in medicine and the improvement of women's health. The site lists women's health books, publications, and provides information about various health topics.

http://www.amwa-doc.org

American Physical Therapy Association

This site offers information for patients and physical therapists alike. Links to other Internet resources and the Amazon Books site provide additional information.

http://www.apta.org

American Telemedicine Association

Established in 1993 as a nonprofit organization and headquartered in Washington, DC, membership in the association is open to individuals, companies, and other organizations with an interest in promoting the deployment of telemedicine throughout the United States and worldwide. The site offers a members-only side and a public side, including a yet to be implemented section on e-health.

http://www.atmeda.org/

The Arthritis Foundation

Extensive information for patients and parents of patients with arthritis. The site contains a large number of links to relevant information and other sites.

http://www.arthritis.org/

Canadian Cancer Society

This is the leading Canadian nonprofit organization focusing on education about cancer prevention and treatment.

http://www.cancer.ca

National Association of Public Hospitals and Health Systems

The National Association of Public Hospitals and Health Systems is an organization that represents the nation's urban public hospitals, health systems, and the people they serve. Its mission is to educate the public and policymakers about the challenges facing public hospitals and the populations they assist. It is an advocate for health care reform that would improve insurance coverage, access to health care, and the general well-being of those who are the most vulnerable participants in the nation's health system.

http://www.naph.org

National Institute on Aging (NIA)

The NIA offers brochures and fact sheets regarding health and aging, including diseases/conditions, health promotion, disease prevention, medical care, medications and immunizations, nutrition, and safety.

http://www.nih.gov/nia/

Nursing World

Nursing World is sponsored by the American Nurses Association and offers links to products, services, journals, continuing education, and more.

http://www.nursingworld.org

Osteoporosis and Related Bone Diseases National Resource Center

This site is your complete source for osteoporosis information including details about Paget's disease of the bone and osteogenesis imperfecta. It's supported by the National Institute of Arthritis and Musculoskeletal and Skin Diseases.

http://www.osteo.org/

Royal College of Physicians and Surgeons of Canada

The Royal College of Physicians and Surgeons of Canada offers this site in both English and French for its members.

http://rcpsc.medical.org/

World Health Organization

The homepage of the World Wide Web InfoServer of WHO, among the UN systems and the major international organizations in Geneva, Switzerland. For comprehensive background information on world health data, this site is invaluable. It includes a *Weekly Epidemiological Record* with access to back copies and a *Statistical Information System* that covers a range of diseases as well as public health categories of risk.

http://www.who.org/

Cancer

American Cancer Society

This site offers local and national cancer news and the ability to search the site for specific content. It includes a media services section that is interesting and a useful source of information for those in the media.

http://www.cancer.org

Canadian Cancer Society

This site is sponsored by the leading Canadian nonprofit organization focusing on education about cancer prevention and treatment.

http://www.cancer.ca

Communicable Disease

Travel Health Online

This online site provides information about travel-related health issues.

http://www.tripprep.com

Computers and Health

American Medical Informatics Association (AMIA)

This is the site of the American Medical Informatics Association (AMIA), a nonprofit membership organization of individuals, institutions, and corporations dedicated to developing and using information technologies to improve health care. The 3200 members of AMIA include physicians, nurses, computer and information scientists, biomedical engineers, medical librarians, and academic researchers and educators.

   http://www.amia.org

Department of Medical Informatics

Here you can find the most relevant links to Web sites on health informatics. Simply choose a country from the index and the links to that particular country will appear.

   http://www.imbi.uni-freiburg.de/medinf/mi_list.htm

MDChoice.com

The former *NetMedicine.com* site, this site offers portals for both patients and physicians.

   http://www.mdchoice.com

Medifor Inc.

This Internet service offers customizable patient education materials to supplement physicians' care instructions on over 800 primary care topics. It offers links to related sites.

   http://www.medifor.com

The Patient Education Institute

The Patient Education Institute offers software and hardware services to health care institutions interested in implementing interactive health communication systems for patient education, informed consent, health promotion, patient satisfaction survey, patient medical history, and service promotion.

   http://www.patient-education.com

History and Reference

Merck Manual (17th edition)

The 17th edition of the famous *Merck Manual* is the centennial edition. It is available online and the site provides search capabilities to make its use easier.

   http://www.merck.com/pubs/mmanual/

Medical Internet Guides

Academic Medicine Events and Meetings

This is a list from the Association of American Medical Colleges.

   http://www.aamc.org/meetings/start.htm

AMA Online CME Locator

This site provides a quick access point to US continuing medical education accredited AMA category I CME providers and activities. Search criteria include the type of CME activity, disease subject area, location by a map of states, dates, faculty, and titles.

http://www.ama-assn.org/cgi-bin/cme-redir

Association of American Medical Colleges

The medical schools and programs are listed alphabetically in order of state or province. It also indicates whether each school participates in the American Medical College Application Service (AMCAS), the University of Texas System Medical and Dental Application Center (UTSM-DAC), or the Ontario Medical School Application Service (OMSAS).

http://www.aamc.org

American Red Cross

Access to information and services provided by the American Red Cross is available here, including health education, health services, blood services, and disaster relief. The site also hosts an extensive "virtual museum" with images and information about the history and development of the American Red Cross.

http://www.redcross.org

Canadian Medical Association Journal

This site contains abstracts from Canada's premier peer-reviewed journal.

http://www.cma.ca/cmaj/index.asp

Canadian Medical Association Journal Index

There are links to more than a dozen journals, newsletters, and reports from the Canadian Medical Association at this site maintained by the CMA.

http://www.cma.ca/publications/index.htm

Doctor's Guide

A doctor's guide to the Internet resources that includes links, news, medical alerts, and a list of conferences and meetings.

http://www.pslgroup.com/MEDRES.HTM

Doctor's Guide to the Internet

The site gives medical news and alerts, new drug advice, medical conference details, publications, and patient information and resources. *Doctor's Guide* was designed to help physicians cost-effectively harness the resources of the Internet and the World Wide Web.

http://www.docguide.com/default.htm

Doctors' Guide to the Internet Medical Meetings

A comprehensive searchable list of medical meetings and conferences organized by category is available through this site.

http://www.pslgroup.com/MEDSITES.HTM

Health Canada Online

Health Canada is the federal department responsible for helping the people of Canada maintain and improve their health. This site offers news and information about health maintenance and specific diseases in either English or French. The site is searchable and contains lots of useful facts such as information for travelers, food guides, and news stories.

http://www.hc-sc.gc.ca/english/

HealthGate Biomedical Databases

This site includes CME, biomedical databases, literature searches, and so on. Free and fee-based services are available.

http://www.healthgate.com

JAMA Homepage — Americal Medical Association

This is a searchable article and abstract collection from *JAMA*. It requires registration.

http://jama.ama-assn.org/

Journal of the American Academy of Orthopaedic Surgeons

This site offers the ability to search and view the table of contents from past issues. Information about the journal and subscriptions are offered as well.

http://www.JAAOS.ORG

The Journal of Bone and Joint Surgery (American Edition)

This site provides access to contents, abstracts, and subscription information.

http://www.jbjs.org

The Lancet

This site offers full-text summaries of selected articles from *Lancet*.

http://www.thelancet.com

Medical Education Online (MEO)

Medical Education Online (MEO) is a forum for disseminating information on educating physicians and other health professionals. Manuscripts on any aspect of the process of training health professionals are considered for peer-reviewed publication in their electronic journal. In addition to manuscripts, *MEO* provides a repository for resources such as curricula, data sets, syllabi, software, and instructional material developers wish to make available to the health education community. The site also posts informational messages and links to World Wide Web sites of interest to health science educators.

http://www.med-ed-online.org

Medical Journal Club on the Web

This is an online, interactive general medical "journal club" that summarizes internal medicine articles from the recent medical literature and appends reader comments.

http://www.webcom.com/mjljweb/jrnlclb/index.html

Medical World Search

Medical World Search is best used for specific clinical searches involving diseases and conditions. The site allows you to search the full text of nearly 100,000 Web pages from thousands of medical sites.

http://www.mwsearch.com

Medscape

Medscape for health professionals and interested consumers, features thousands of full-text, peer-reviewed articles, medical news, MEDLINE, and interactive quizzes.

http://www.medscape.com/default.mhtml

National Women's Health Resource Center

This site is quite possibly the leading US federal clearinghouse for women's health information.

http://www.healthywomen.org/

New England Journal of Medicine Online

Extended abstracts and limited full text are available here from the *New England Journal*.

http://www.nejm.org/content/index.asp

Physicians' News Digest

This is a comprehensive database of continuing medical education programs searchable by topic, date, sponsor, and location.

http://www.physiciansnews.com/cme.html

PubMed

This is NLM's search service to access the 9 million citations in *MEDLINE* and *Pre-MEDLINE* (with links to participating online journals), and other related databases.

http://www.ncbi.nlm.nih.gov/PubMed/

The Residency Page

The site lists all known medical residencies.

http://www.residencysite.com

The US National Library of Medicine

This is the entry point for the National Library of Medicine including general information, databases, and photographic archives. Connections to comprehensive databases of medical information such as *MEDLARS* and *MEDLINE* are also available.

http://www.nlm.nih.gov/

WebMedLit

This site provides efficient access to the best medical journals on the Web. It currently tracks 18 medical journals, and allows you to view the latest medical literature on the Web by topic. This site is a service of Web Medical Literature Services.

http://www.webmedlit.com/

Medical News and Information

NLM National Telemedicine Initiative

This is the National Library of Medicine's site dealing with various aspects of the National Telemedicine Initiative. There is information about the initiative, projects supported by the initiative, up-coming meetings, and more.

http://www.nlm.nih.gov/research/telemedinit.html

Telemedicine Information Exchange

The *Telemedicine Information Exchange* was created and is maintained by the Telemedicine Research Center with major support from the National Library of Medicine. This site is a comprehensive, international, quality-filtered resource for information about telemedicine and telemedicine-related activities.

http://tie.telemed.org/

Medical Publishers

Audio Digest Foundation

The Audio Digest Foundation has provided medical professionals throughout the world with continuing medical education on audio tape since 1954. Its Web site offers a chance to view current topics and place orders.

http://www.audio-digest.org/

Blackwell North America Core Publisher List

This site is based on entries in the *Blackwell Approval Publishers List* and supplemented by *Literary Market Place* and the *Association of American University Presses Directory*.

http://www.blackwell.com/shelf/tools/cormed.htm

Krames Communications

This site is sponsored by the publisher of consumer-oriented information on medical, wellness, and injury prevention topics.

http://www.krames.com

Lippincott Williams & Wilkins Publishers

The site contains information about books, electronic media, and periodicals. The site offers a search engine and online ordering capabilities as well.

http://www.lww.com/

Medical Association Communications

Sponsored by the publisher for medical associations, meeting highlights, and online medical journals, the site provides medical professionals with *Highlights* from annual meetings of a number of medical associations, and selected continuing education programs in print and CD-ROM. Excerpts of full proceedings can be downloaded, or the original document or disk can be ordered at no cost.

http://www.macmcm.com/

Harcourt Health

Harcourt is the world's leading publisher of books, journals, and serial publications in the health sciences—medicine, nursing, allied health sciences, dentistry, veterinary medicine—and selected college disciplines—health, physical education and recreation, nutrition, and chemistry. Its WWW page has *What's New at Harcourt* this month, a large catalog of health-sciences texts, videos, and software, and information about conferences and seminars that are currently being offered.

http://www.harcourthealth.com/Mosby/index.html

Springer-Verlag

The site offers a searchable catalog of information and publications in the fields of biology and biomedicine, chemistry, computer science, economics and law, engineering, ecology and environmental sciences, geoscience, mathematics, medicine, physics and astronomy, psychology, and statistics.

http://www.springer-ny.com/

Thieme Medical Publishers

This is the site of the book and journal publisher in the fields of neurosurgery, audiology, ophthalmology, orthopaedics, otolaryngology, radiology, dentistry, and complementary medicine.

http://www.thieme.com/

Pharmaceuticals and Products

The Internet FDA

The Food and Drug Administration site offers information to consumers and health professionals on a wide variety of its activities.

http://www.fda.gov/

New Drugs List

A listing of new drugs, including chemical and trade names, a brief description, and manufacturer.

http://cctr.umkc.edu/user/mash/newdrugs.html

PDR for Physicians

Presented by Medical Economics (the publisher of the printed version), this site offers the *Physicians' Desk Reference (PDR)* as well as the *PDR* for herbal medications and *PDR* for multiple drug interactions. Other options include access to new drug and pricing information.

http://physician.pdr.net/physician/index.htm

Physiotherapy

American Physical Therapy Association

This site offers information for patients and physical therapists alike. Links to other Internet resources and the Amazon Books site provide additional information.

http://www.apta.org

Practice Management

Mednetrix.com

This company offers to help develop a Web site for you that is customized to an individual medical practice and its medical specialty. You control the content.

http://www.mednetrix.com

Medscape

Medscape offers an electronic record system that includes digital health records, and allows access anytime and anywhere a physician–patient encounter takes place. As of June, 2000, more than 13 million patient records had been created with its system. This site gives overviews of the system and a demonstration.

http://www.medicalogic.com

General Interest

Fitness and Exercise

The Fitness Jumpsite

This is a Web site that proclaims that it wants to be "your connection to a lifestyle of fitness, nutrition, and health." It contains information and links to fitness and lifestyle issues. A great little grassroots site (read: noncommercial labor of love) providing extensive links and content for the fitness-minded, along with support for people struggling to lose weight or otherwise get in shape. This everything-to-everyone resource also lets you investigate a new sport, search reviews of sports equipment, or browse hundreds of links to other Web sites.

http://www.primusweb.com/fitnesspartner/

FitnessZone's Fitness Profile

The site contains an easy-to-complete fitness assessment that helps calculate your target workout heart rate, and gives advice on general fitness goals. It provides you with a detailed fitness profile, including overall fitness rating and nutrition and exercise plans, and recommends a pace for you to exercise, based on this profile.

http://www.fitnesszone.com/profiles/

Fitness Online

This is a cool site with advice on fitness, training, and nutrition. It provides links to 'zines including *Shape*, *Muscle and Fitness*, *Flex*, and *Men's Fitness*.

http://www.fitnessonline.com/

Male Health Center

The site provides a wide variety of information regarding many aspects of the male species.

http://www.malehealthcenter.com/

MEDic Men's Health Issues

Info and research on various men's health issues is available here.

http://medic.med.uth.tmc.edu/ptnt/00000391.htm

The Health Mall: Health, Nutrition, Fitness, and Personal Development

The Health Mall is both a resource center and shopping mall featuring businesses that offer products, services, and information related to health, nutrition, fitness, and personal development. Some stores are strictly informational; others offer online ordering; some offer coupons. The mall

includes a searchable database of health food stores in the US, an online magazine called *A Healthy Day*, a classified section, and a resource center.
http://www.hlthmall.com

Shape Up America!

Designed to provide the latest information about safe weight management and physical fitness, the site includes keyword and concept searches.
http://www.shapeup.org/

Women's Health Interactive

Women's Health Interactive's mission is to create a learning environment where multidisciplinary health education resources are accessible to women and health care professionals. The National Women's Health Resource Center provides the site with *What's Hot in Women's Health!*, health updates from its award-winning publication, the *National Women's Health Report*.
http://www.womens-health.com

Living and Lifestyle

Amazon.com

Billed as the largest online bookstore, it has made shopping and ordering so easy that 4.5 million customers have already bought books, music, and more. You can search for titles, subjects, or areas of interest in books, music, CDs, DVDs, and gifts. From browsing to serious shopping, with over 3 million titles, if you can't find it here you may want to rethink your needs.
http://www.Amazon.com

Barnes and Noble Booksellers

Online book shopping at this megastore is easy. From just wandering about, to bargain bins, to online chats with current authors, the site has something for most avid bibliophiles. If you are not quite ready to do your shopping online, the site includes the opportunity to find the location of your nearest store by entering your zip code.
http://www.barnesandnoble.com/

CDC Travel Information

This comprehensive guide to health-related travel information is maintained by the Centers for Disease Control and Prevention. It includes information about geographic health recommendations and current disease outbreaks.
http://www.cdc.gov/travel

CNN Interactive

From breaking news to wire service stories, the CNN site gives you access to news and information almost as it happens. The site contains clickable headings such as world, United States, politics, weather, business, sports, science and technology, entertainment, books, travel, health, and others. There is even an option to customize the news you receive.

http://www.cnn.com/

CNN—Sports Illustrated

For sports fans of all sorts, this site can give you minute-by-minute scores, recaps, and feature stories, audio and video, and more. (I don't know if it carries the swimsuit issue.)

http://sportsillustrated.cnn.com/

CNNFN—The Financial Network

This is the financial cousin of the CNN site and provides ample business news and information for even the most dedicated stock watcher.

http://cnnfn.cnn.com/

CollegeBound Network

This is another excellent site for students and parents facing the process of college selection, application, and matriculation.

http://collegebound.net

International Travelers Clinic

The Medical College of Wisconsin International Travelers Clinic located at Froedtert Hospital provides comprehensive preventive health care services for travelers planning trips abroad. The site provides lots of health information important for the international traveler.

http://www.intmed.mcw.edu/travel.html

Lycos Maps

At this site you can type in the street or address you want to find and get a custom-drawn map. This site is great if you are traveling to unfamiliar places near or far. You can enter any two addresses and get directions, driving distance and time, and a map, all in a matter of seconds. If you want to get fancy, you can enter a telephone number and have the site tell you where the call came from.

http://maps.lycos.com

The New York Times

News as well as classifieds, arts, restaurants, and more are here at the electronic version of "All the news that's fit...."

http://www.nytimes.com

SmartMoney.com

The *SmartMoney* site provides access to a number of financial planning tools and information resources.

http://www.smartmoney.com

Time.com

This site is an interesting mixture of articles and features from the wide array of Time-Warner periodicals, including *Time*, *Money*, *Fortune*, *Mutual Funds*, *People*, and *Entertainment Weekly*. Also links to *Zagat's Restaurant Review* on the Web and much more.

http://www.time.com/time/index.html

The Washington Post

Here is a chance to follow what is being said in one of the country's most influential papers. The site includes features such as *Today's Edition* and *Yesterday's Edition* so when people are discussing something in the paper and you didn't have time to stop and buy it, you can go back to the site and look!

http://www.washingtonpost.com

The Weather Channel

The Weather Channel homepage provides weather information for anywhere in the world. This can be useful when planning trips to meetings. It also provides medically related information such as pollen maps and information about colds and flu.

http://www.weather.com

United Parcel Service

The UPS site allows you to calculate transit times and track shipments online—helpful when you are expecting that package from eBay.

http://www.ups.com/

USA Today

It is only logical that a paper that is composed and published almost exclusively by electronic means should be on the Web. The site offers the usual news and information, but is particularly strong in sports and weather information, a real help when traveling.

http://www.usatoday.com

Whowhere

This is a portal to a number of sites that can help you locate almost anyone in the United States.

http://www.whowhere.lycos.com/

Appendix 3
Departments of Orthopaedic Surgery: Domestic and International

United States

Alabama
   University of Alabama Medical Center Program
      http://www.ortho.uab.edu
   University of South Alabama Program
      http://www.southalabama.edu/

Arizona
   Maricopa Medical Center Program
      http://phoenixorthoresident.com
   University of Arizona Program
      http://www.bones.arizona.edu

Arkansas
   University of Arkansas for Medical Sciences Program
      http://www.uams.edu/ortho/ortho.htm

California
   Loma Linda University Program
      http://www.llu.edu/llumc/residency.html
   UCLA Medical Center Program
      http://149.142.183.2
   University of Southern California/LAC+USC Medical
      Center Program
      http://www.usc.edu/medicine/orthopaedic_surgery
   University of California (Irvine) Program
      http://www.ucihs.uci.edu/ortho
   University of California (Davis) Health System Program
      http://www.ucdmc.ucdavis.edu/departments/ortho.html
   University of California (San Diego) Program
      http://medicine.ucsd.edu/ortho

San Francisco Program
   http://www.sforp.com
University of California (San Francisco) Program
   http://www.ucsf.edu/orthopedics
Stanford University Program
   http://www.med.stanford.edu/shc/ortho/residency.html
Los Angeles County-Harbor-UCLA Medical Center Program
   http://www.careermd.com

Colorado
   University of Colorado Program
      http://www.uchsc.edu/sm/ortho/resdcy.html

Connecticut
   University of Connecticut Program
      http://uconnortho.uchc.edu/wwwdocdb/
   Yale–New Haven Medical Center Program
      http://www.info.med.yale.edu/ortho/

District of Columbia
   Georgetown University Program
      http://www.dml.georgetown.edu/hospital/housestaff/
   George Washington University Program
      http://www.gwumc.edu/edu/ortho

Florida
   University of Florida Program
      http://www.med.ufl.edu/ortho
   University of Florida Health Science Center/Jacksonville Program
      http://www.ufl.edu
   Jackson Memorial Hospital/Jackson Health System Program
      http://www.miami.edu/ortho
   Orlando Regional Healthcare System Program
      http://www.orhs.org

Georgia
   Emory University Program
      http://www.emory.edu/WHSC/ORTHO
   Atlanta Medical Center Program
      http://www.amc-gme.com
   Medical College of Georgia Program
      http://www.mcg.edu/resident/ortho/index.html

Hawaii
   University of Hawaii Program
      http://hawaiiresidency.org
   Tripler Army Medical Center Program
      http://www.tamc.amedd.army.mil

Illinois
   University of Chicago Program
      http://www.chicagoorthopaedics.com
   Rush-Presbyterian-St Luke's Medical Center Program
      http://www.rush.edu
   McGaw Medical Center of Northwestern University Program
      http://www.orthopaedics.nwu.edu
   University of Illinois College of Medicine at Chicago Program
      http://www.uic.edu/com/ors
   Loyola University Program
      http://www.luhs.org/under/specserv/orthopae.htm
   Southern Illinois University Program
      http://www.siumed.edu/education/residency/ortho.html

Indiana
   Fort Wayne Medical Education Program
      http://www.fwmep.edu
   Indiana University School of Medicine Program
      http://www.iupui.edu/it/iuortho/orthohome.html

Iowa
   University of Iowa Hospitals and Clinics Program
      http://www.medicine.uiowa.edu/ortho

Kansas
   University of Kansas Medical Center Program
      http://www2.kumc.edu/ortho/surg.htm
   University of Kansas (Wichita) Program
      http://wichita.kumc.edu/ortho/

Kentucky
   University of Kentucky Medical Center Program
      http://www.uky.edu/surgery
   University of Louisville Program
      http://www.louisville.edu/medschool/orthos

Louisiana

Louisiana State University Program
http://www.lsuhsc.edu
Tulane University Program
http://www.mcl.tulane.edu/departments/orthopaedics
Alton Ochsner Medical Foundation Program
http://www.ochsner.org/dome/gmeweb/index.htm
Louisiana State University (Shreveport) Program
http://www.ortho.lsuhsc.edu/

Maryland

Johns Hopkins University Program
http://www.med.jhu.edu/ortho/
Union Memorial Hospital Program
http://www.unionmemorial.org
University of Maryland Program
http://www.umm.edu/surg-ortho/

Massachusetts

Massachusetts General Hospital/Harvard Medical School Program
http://www.healthcare.partners.org/harvardorthoweb
Boston University Medical Center Program
http://www.bumc.bu.edu/orthopaedics
University of Massachusetts Program
http://www.umassmed.edu/orthopedics/residency

Michigan

University of Michigan Program
http://www.med.umich.edu/surg/ortho
Wayne State University/Detroit Medical Center Program
http://www.uortho.com
McLaren Regional Medical Center Program
http://www.McLaren.org
Grand Rapids Medical Education and Research Center/ Michigan State University Program
http://www.bone.net
Kalamazoo Center for Medical Studies/Michigan State University Program
http://www.kcms.msu.edu/programs/orthopaedic
William Beaumont Hospital Program
http://www.beaumont.edu/gme

Minnesota
  University of Minnesota Program
    http://www.ortho.umn.edu
  Mayo Graduate School of Medicine (Rochester) Program
    http://www.mayo.edu/

Missouri
  University of Missouri-Columbia Program
    http://www.muhealth.org/~ortho/
  University of Missouri at Kansas City Program
    http://ortho.umkc.edu
  St Louis University School of Medicine Program
    http://medschool.slu.edu/orthosurg
  Washington University/B-JH/SLCH Consortium Program
    http://www.ortho.wustl.edu

Nebraska
  University of Nebraska/Creighton University Program
    http://www.unmc.edu/orthosurgery/

New Hampshire
  Dartmouth-Hitchcock Medical Center Program
    http://www.hitchcock.org/pages/GME/Ortho.htm

New Jersey
  Monmouth Medical Center Program
    http://www.saintbarnabas.com/education/mmced/index.html
  UMDNJ-Robert Wood Johnson Medical School Program
    http://www2.umdnj.edu/orthoweb/chief.htm
  UMDNJ-New Jersey Medical School Program
    http://www.umdnj.edu/orthnweb/

New Mexico
  University of New Mexico Program
    http://hsc.unm.edu/ortho

New York
  Albany Medical Center Program
    http://www.amc.edu/GME/orthopaedic_surgery_residency.htm
  SUNY Health Science Center at Brooklyn Program
    http://www.downstate.edu
  Albert Einstein College of Medicine at Long Island Jewish Medical
    Center Program

http://www.lij.edu
Mount Sinai School of Medicine Program
  http://www.mssm.edu/orthopaedics/
Hospital for Special Surgery/Cornell Medical Center Program
  http://www.hss.edu
New York University Medical Center/Hospital for Joint Diseases Orthopaedic Institute Program
  http://www.hjd.edu
University of Rochester Program
  http://www.urmc.rochester.edu
SUNY Upstate Medical University Program
  http://www.upstate.edu/ortho/

North Carolina
  University of North Carolina Hospitals Program
    http://www.med.unc.edu/ortho
  Duke University Program
    http://surgery.mc.duke.edu/orthopaedics
  Wake Forest University School of Medicine Program
    http://www.wfubmc.edu/ortho

Ohio
  Summa Health System/NEOUCOM Program
    http://www.summahealth.org/edu
  Akron General Medical Center/NEOUCOM Program
    http://www.akrongeneral.org
  University Hospital/University of Cincinnati College of Medicine Program
    http://www.uc.edu/orthopaedics/
  Cleveland Clinic Foundation Program
    http://www.ccf.org/education/fellows/ors.htm
  Ohio State University Program
    http://www.ortho.ohio-state.edu/
  Mount Carmel Program
    http://www.mountcarmelhealth.com/medicaleducation/gme
  Wright State University Program
    http://www.med.wright.edu/ortho/res
  Medical College of Ohio Program
    http://mco.edu

Oklahoma
  University of Oklahoma Health Sciences Center Program
    http://w3.ouhsc.edu/orthopedics

Orgeon
    Oregon Health & Science University Program
        http://www.ohsu.edu/som-Orthopedics

Pennsylvania
    Geisinger Medical Center Program
        http://www.geisinger.edu
    Hamot Medical Center Program
        http://www.hamot.org
    Penn State University/Milton S. Hershey Medical Center Program
        http://www.hmc.psu.edu/orthopaedics/residency/index.htm
    Albert Einstein Medical Center Program
        http://www.einstein.edu/phl/1225.html
    University of Pennsylvania Program
        http://www.med.upenn.edu/ortho/
    MCP Hahnemann University Program
        http://www.mcphu.edu/medschool/residency/OrthoSurg.html
    Temple University Program
        http://www.temple.edu/orthopaedics/index.html
    Thomas Jefferson University Program
        http://www.tjuhortho.org
    University Health Center of Pittsburgh Program
        http://www.orthonet.upmc.edu
    Allegheny General Hospital Program
        http://www.wpahs.org

Rhode Island
    Brown University Program
        http://biomed.brown.edu/medicine_departments/orthopaedics/
        defaul

South Carolina
    Medical University of South Carolina Program
        http://www.musc.edu/orthosurg
    Palmetto Health Alliance/University of South Carolina School of Med-
    icine Program
        http://www.palmettohealth.com/residency/
    Greenville Hospital System Program
        http://www.ghs.org

Tennessee
    University of Tennessee College of Medicine at Chattanooga Program
        http://www.erlanger.org/utcom/orthopaedic.html

University of Tennessee Program
http://www.utmem.edu/ortho/homepage.html
Vanderbilt University Program
http://www.mc.vanderbilt.edu/ortho

Texas
University of Texas Southwestern Medical School Program
http://www.swmed.edu/home_pages/OrthoSurg
San Antonio Uniformed Services Health Education Consortium
(BAMC) Program
http://www.gprmc.amedd.army.mil/bamc/ortho.htm
John Peter Smith Hospital (Tarrant County Hospital District)
Program
http://www.jpshealthnet.org
University of Texas Medical Branch Hospitals Program
http://www.utmb.edu/ortho
University of Texas at Houston Program
http://www.ortho1.med.uth.tmc.edu/newpage/ut.htm
Baylor College of Medicine Program
http://public.bcm.tmc.edu/departments/ortho.html
Texas Tech University (Lubbock) Program
http://www.ttuhsc.edu/pages/ortho/welcome.htm
University of Texas Health Science Center at San Antonio Program
http://www.uthscsa.edu/orthopaedics/
San Antonio Uniformed Services Health Education Consortium
(WHMC) Program
http://www.whmc.af.mil
Texas A&M College of Medicine–Scott and White Program
http://www.sw.org

Utah
University of Utah Program
http://www.med.utah.edu/orthopedics

Virginia
University of Virginia Program
http://www.med.va.edu/medicine/clinical/orthopaedics
Naval Medical Center (Portsmouth) Program
http://www.nmcp.med.navy.mil/ortho/orthohome.htm

Vermont
University of Vermont Program
http://www.vtmednet.org/~g136911

Washington
  University of Washington Program
    http://www.orthop.washington.edu/
  Madigan Army Medical Center Program
    http://www.mamc.amedd.army.mil/gme/index.htm

West Virginia
  West Virginia University Program
    http://www.hsc.wvu.edu./som/orthopedics.html

Wisconsin
  University of Wisconsin Program
    http://www.mcw.edu/ortho/
  Medical College of Wisconsin Program
    http://www.mcw.edu/ortho

International

Institute of Orthopaedics at The Robert Jones and Agnes Hunt Oswestry Shropshire United Kingdom

The Institute of Orthopaedics is the research and teaching unit of the Robert Jones and Agnes Hunt Orthopaedic and District Hospital NHS Trust.
  http://www.keele.ac.uk/depts/rjah/rjah.htm

University of Vienna — Department of Trauma

The homepage of Universitätsklinik für Unfallchirurgie Universität Wien.
  http://www.akh-wien.ac.at/trauma/

Biomechanics Lab, Istituti Ortopedici Rizzoli, Bologna, Italy

The homepage of the Biomechanics Laboratory, Istituti Ortopedici Rizzoli, via di Barbiano 1/10, 40136 Bologna, Italy.
  http://www.ior.it/biomec/

Carleton University Sports Medicine Clinic, Ottawa, Ontario, Canada

The homepage of Carleton University Sports Medicine Clinic.
  http://www.carletonsportsmed.com/front.htm

Chinese University of Hong Kong Department of Orthopaedics Traumatology

The homepage of the Chinese University of Hong Kong Department of Orthopaedics & Traumatology.
  http://www.cuhk.edu.hk/med/ort/med_ort.htm

Chinese University of Hong Kong Orthopaedic Learning Centre

Orthopaedic Learning Centre, CUHK.
  http://www.olc.ort.cuhk.edu.hk/index.htm

Dalhousie Orthopaedic Surgery

Dalhousie Medical School is based in Halifax, Nova Scotia, and is the only medical school in Maritime Canada.

http://www.medicine.dal.ca/dortho/

Department of Hand Surgery at St. James's University Hospital

The homepage of the Department of Hand Surgery at St. James's University Hospital, Leeds, UK.

http://www.leeds.ac.uk/handsurgery/

Dundee University Distance Learning

Orthopaedic & Trauma Surgery.

http://www.dundee.ac.uk/Orthopaedics/dls/dls.htm

Edinburgh Orthopaedic Trauma Unit

The homepage of the Edinburgh Orthopaedic Trauma Unit.

http://www.trauma.co.uk/

Edinburgh University Department of Orthopaedic Surgery

The Edinburgh University Department of Orthopaedic Surgery encompasses one of the longest established orthopaedic and trauma centers in the United Kingdom.

http://www.orthopaedic.ed.ac.uk

European Paediatric Orthopaedic Society

The homepage of the European Paediatric Orthopaedic Surgery.

http://www.cilea.it/ortopedia/

Flinders University of South Australia

http://www.flinders.edu.au/

Fowler Kennedy Sports Medicine Clinic, London, Ontario, Canada

http://www.fowlerkennedy.com/

Hillerød Sygehus Department of Orthopaedic Surgery, Denmark

HIS Ortopaedkirurgisk Afdeling O.

http://www.fa.dk/sundhed/A-SYGEHU/HILLEROD/10-ORT-O/4-ORTOP.htm

Institute of Orthopaedic Research and Biomechanics, Ulm, Germany

The homepage of the Institute for Orthopaedic Research and Biomechanics, Ulm.

http://lyra.medizin.uni-ulm.de/ufb.html/ufb-home.html surgery.html

Maurice E. Müller Institute for Biomechanics, Switzerland

Orthopaedic Biomechanics Division (OBD).

http://cranium.unibe.ch/

McGill Division of Orthopaedic Surgery, Canada

McGill Ortho Site.
http://ww2.mcgill.ca/orthopaedics/

McGill University, Montreal, Quebec, Canada

The homepage of McGill University.
http://www.mcgill.ca/

Nuffield Orthopaedic Surgery Oxford

The homepage of the Nuffield Department of Orthopaedic Surgery.
http://www.ox.ac.uk/cgi-bin/contact/newaceunits?ortho

OrthoNet University of Toronto

OrthoNet was initially developed to serve the needs of residents in the Orthopaedic Surgery program at the University of Toronto. However, over time *OrthoNet* has evolved into a Web portal for orthopaedic residents across Canada and abroad.
http://www.orthonet.on.ca/

Orthopädische Universitätsklinik Bochum am St. Anna-Hospital, Germany

Startseite.
http://www.ruhr-uni-bochum.de/annaherne/

Queens University, Ontario, Canada, Division of Orthopaedic Surgery

Division of Orthopaedic Surgery.
http://meds.queensu.ca/medicine/ortho/

Service d'Orthopédie et de Traumatologie de l'appareil locomoteur Bruxelles, Belgique

Service d'Orthopédie et de Traumatologie de l'Appareil Locomoteur.
http://www.md.ucl.ac.be/entites/chir/orto/intro.htm

Surgical Medical Research Institute, University of Alberta

Surgical Medical Research Institute.
http://www.ualberta.ca/~smri/SMRI.htm

Trauma Program

Sunnybrook and Women's College Health Sciences Centre.
http://www.sunnybrookandwomens.on.ca/programs/section.cfm?d

Université Catholique de Louvain (Catholic University of Leu), Belgium

UCL—Administration centrale (AC).
http://www.ac.ucl.ac.be

University Hospital Pellenberg Department of Orthopaedics Katholieke Universiteit Leuven, Belgium

Welcome to the Department of Orthopaedics University Hospital Pellenberg.
http://www.belgianorthoweb.be/pellenberg/index.htm

University of Antwerpen

The homepage of the Universiteit Antwerpen.
  http://www.ua.ac.be/index.html

University of Calgary

The homepage of the University of Calgary, Alberta, Canada.
  http://www.ucalgary.ca

University of Dundee

The homepage of the University of Dundee.
  http://www.dundee.ac.uk/

University of Dundee Orthopaedic and Trauma Surgery

The homepage of the University of Dundee Orthopaedic and Trauma
Surgery.
  http://www.dundee.ac.uk/Orthopaedics/

University of Edinburgh

The homepage of the University of Edinburgh, promoting excellence in
teaching and research.
  http://www.ed.ac.uk/

University of Manitoba, Section of Orthopaedics

The homepage of the University of Manitoba Department of Surgery.
  http://www.umanitoba.ca/faculties/medicine/units/surgery/

University of Queensland

Access information about the University of Queensland, its faculties,
schools, and the programs it offers.
  http://www.uq.oz.au/

University of Sheffield

The homepage of the University of Sheffield, United Kingdom.
  http://www2.shef.ac.uk/

University of Toronto

The homepage of the University of Toronto.
  http://www.utoronto.ca/uoft.html

University of Ulm

The homepage of the Hauptseite der Universität Ulm.
  http://www.uni-ulm.de/

University of Western Ontario Faculty of Medicine and Dentistry

The homepage of the University of Western Ontario.
  http://www.med.uwo.ca/

Glossary of Terms

Address
The location of an Internet resource such as a Web site (URL) or the e-mail address for personal contact of an individual.

Address book
Part of the e-mail program, that stores the names and e-mail addresses of your correspondents. Some viruses are designed to read your address book and replicate themselves by sending infected messages to everyone in it.

Always-on connection
This refers to the DSL (digital subscriber line) or cable modem line that is always connected. This is a high-speed connection that does not require the user to dial up the connection on a modem. It is "always connected" and a click on the icon of the browser will display the World Wide Web.

AOL
America Online. The largest provider of Internet service, with e-mail, chat rooms, instant messaging, and an Internet connection.

Applet
A JAVA program (little application) that is loaded with a Web page to produce some more complex form of display or interaction.

Application
A program that runs on your computer to undertake useful work (or play). In contrast, system programs undertake functions relating to the workings of your computer.

ASCII
American Standard Code for Information Interchange. This is the basic analogue text file used on the Internet

Binary file
The digital file composed of 1s and 0s that is used on the Internet for images and video transfer.

Binary number
A number is either on or off (1 or 0 for clarity). The computer has no shades of meaning for that piece of information. This is what contributes to the accuracy of computers: the fundamental information cannot be confused. If you string binary numbers together, you

can get larger numbers. For example, the binary number 1001 translates as 1 one, no twos, no fours, and 1 eight, total 9.

BMP file This is the standard windows image uncompressed image file.

Browser The software program that interprets and displays the HTML pages of a Web site.

Bug A logic error in a program that results in the program failing. The problem is in the instructions written into the program and cannot be altered by the user (see Patch).

Bugfix The strategy used to eliminate a bug from a program.

Byte The unit of storage for computer data. One byte will store an 8-digit binary number (i.e., a number between 0 and 255 decimal). Storage size is usually reckoned in kilobytes, megabytes, or gigabytes.

Client computer The computer on the receiving end of file transfer, usually the computer being used to access information. By contrast the file server or host computer is the one that stores the files and sends them on demand.

Default The file or program used whenever the choice is not specified. For example, the actual file required for loading to your browser is not specified when you give the address **http://owl.orthogate.com.** The default file is opened (**http://owl.orthogate.com/Default.htm**). The OS also uses defaults so that, for example, it will open a Web page in the default browser program when you click on a link from any program except another browser. Defaults are also set up for e-mail, Web page editing, image editing, media playing, and a host of other programs. You may need to alter the defaults if you find that a program will not invoke the program you want.

Domain The part of the Internet designated by a unique address. The domain name is the set of words used in the URL to make the address recognizable (like **www.aana.org**). The domain suffix is the end portion of the address of a Web site such as .com, .org, .edu, or regional suffixes such as .ca.

DOS Disk operating system. This is a set of instructions to the computer that govern the way files stored on the computer are accessed, moved, indexed, and generally organized. The adoption of Microsoft DOS (MS-DOS) as the standard operating system for IBM PCs was the foundation of Bill Gates' success.

DSL   Digital Subscriber Line. A fast, always-on connection using telephone lines. Competitive with cable and much faster than the standard modem.

E-mail   Electronic mail. The system whereby messages and attached files can be sent point-to-point across the Internet. Each user of the Internet has a unique e-mail address.

Ethernet   The standard of networking that allows the connection of several computers over a network.

Firewall   This is a hardware device that prevents access to a computer or series of computers via a phone line, cable, or Ethernet line.

Frames   A specific HTML convention that allows the Web designer to separate different parts of the screen. This means that you can change one part without changing all the others. Typically this is used so that a navigation "page" is at the top or to the side of the screen and the content window (frame) is in the center. Clicking in the navigation frame then changes the content frame but the navigation area remains the same.

Front Page   The same as Home Page. FrontPage is also the name of a popular WYSIWYG Web page editor.

FTP   File transfer protocol. The process of transferring files from one computer directly to another over the Internet.

GIF file   Graphics interface file. This still-image Internet format is designed for drawings and graphics with large areas of solid colors.

Hack   To hack into a computer means gaining illegal entry into another computer.

Hardware   The mechanical parts of a computer—chips, circuits, keyboard, mouse, monitor, printer, scanner, etc. (cf. Software).

HIS   Hospital (or health) information system. The computer system that undertakes patient information and other management functions in the hospital. By extension it means the people in the HIS department.

Home Page   The part of the Web site displayed when you first arrive on a site. Good home pages offer a description of the information offered on the site, and rapid navigation to the part of the site that may interest you (see also Splash page). Also, the page that your browser program will open automatically when you start the program. This can be defined in Edit/Preferences (Netscape) or Tools/Internet Options (IE).

Host computer   The computer that stores the information files that a client computer may request.

HTML   Hypertext Markup Language. This is the language of the Internet that is read by a browser. It allows for linking, by underlining words or sentences, to other Web pages. This layering allows complex linking to other pages within the same site or to remote pages on another site.

HTTP   Hypertext Transfer Protocol. This identifies the hypertext file.

Hyperlink   See Link.

Hypertext   A document that goes beyond text, usually containing images and links to other documents. Thus a hypertext document or collection of documents can be viewed by different users in different ways.

Internet   The complex connection of computers around the world.

Internet software   This is software that translates the HTML page to look like a normal word-processor page. Examples of Internet software are the browsers such as Internet Explorer and Netscape.

Intranet   The connection of local computers within an office or business. This may or may not have a connection to the outside Internet.

IS   Information systems. This also refers to the department or group of employees in a business that maintains the computers and their connection to the LAN or Internet.

ISDN   Integrated Services Digital Network. These connections are all digital and avoid the necessity of digital-to-analog conversion that occurs with phone lines and slows things down.

ISP   Internet service provider. The commercial company that owns and maintains the computer that the user

	dials into to gain access to the Internet. The company charges a fee for this service.
IT	Information technology. In the modern context IT denotes computer systems for managing data and information. In its widest sense information technology would include bookshelves, etc.
JAVA	The platform-independent programming language used to create specific subprograms that function within a Web page.
Javascript	JAVA instructions that can be embedded in an HTML page.
JPEG file	Joint Photographic Expert Group. A still-image compressed file for pictures. This format is more suitable for Web use as it is a smaller file size that downloads quickly compared to BMP or TIFF files. The JPEG is the standard for photos that have sharp edges compared to the GIF that is better for graphics with large solid colors.
Keyword list	A section of the heading of an HTML page, usually invisible to the reader, that contains keywords provided by the creator of the Web page to attract search engines. In HTML this list has the format ⟨META NAME="keywords" CONTENT="orthopaedic, orthopedic, surgery"⟩ where the keywords are separated by commas.
LAN	Local area network. A connection between two or more computers. This connection may just involve a small group of computers in an office without connection to the Internet. The LAN may be hardwired or wireless to provide the client with mobility about the home or office.
Link or Hyperlink	An element on a Web page that can direct your browser program to display a new page. The most common convention is that links are blue underlined words, but links may also be images and may be any color or format. The universal way to recognize a link on a Web page is that the cursor changes (usually to a little hand) when it is over a link. Clicking the left mouse button when this occurs results in control being transferred to the new address. Jumping from link to link without absorbing much from any one site is called surfing.

Link rot The process by which links to other pages on the Internet become gradually useless. Because pages are withdrawn or moved to a new address, the address you may be directed to from an unmaintained page may be out of date.

Mac The Macintosh computer produced by Apple, especially the early versions. The Mac operating system was a user-friendly system of popup windows and icons.

Mirror or A Web site that is an exact copy of another site. Mir-
mirror site rors are used when the traffic on a single site may get too heavy for the servers or for security if one of the sites goes down for some reason.

Modem The hardware that connects a computer through a telephone line to a network.

MSN Microsoft Network. An Internet portal developed by Microsoft.

Netiquette The rules of the Internet. This would include not using capital letters in typing, as this is similar to SHOUTING.

Newbie A person who is new to the Internet. There are a number of rules that one should learn before jumping into an Internet discussion group.

On-the-fly Computer actions, such as the preparation of an HTML file, that take place between the request for the information and the serving of the resulting file. On-the-fly files are created from a database and are used when the information is rapidly changing.

OS Operating system. Typically this is Microsoft Windows. The other main contender is the Mac OS. A free OS is Linux, but it is generally used by computer experts.

Page or The display in a browser program, usually text and
Web page graphics. In simple sites this page will be the result of a single file, but sites that use frames may use more than one file per page.

Patch Some computer programming code produced by the manufacturer to add on to a program you are using already. The patch is used to fix a bug in the program or close a loophole that might be exploited by virus designers.

PC Personal computer. The original IBM computer allowed other companies to make clone computers that became known as PCs to distinguish them from the Mac or Apple computers.

PDA   Personal digital assistant. Handheld computers suited to note making, calendars, and an increasing variety of medical applications.

PDF files   A proprietary file format used by Adobe to encode files that can be read over any computer operating system using the Adobe Acrobat Reader software.

Pixel   A picture element or dot of information on the computer screen that produces an image. The more pixels the greater the resolution of the photo.

Platform   The hardware on which a particular application is being run. Typical platforms would be PCs, Macs, PDAs, Linux, etc. Each platform has its own operating system and machine language. As a result many applications are "platform specific"; they can only be run on certain machines.

POP   Point of presence. The common method of connecting from an ISP to an individual user. Access to the Internet is provided by assigning a temporary address to the user.

PowerPoint   Microsoft's Presentation Graphics program in which you can create "slides" to illustrate a presentation. Since the presentation is computer-guided it can contain animated graphics, sound, and video clips. Corel Presentation Graphics is similar.

PPV   Pay per view. WWW Pages that can only be viewed by subscribers or by paying a fee. Many journals have posted their content as PPV.

Prodigy   A commercial Internet service provider that provides a portal of entry to the Internet.

Router   A piece of hardware that shunts information around on the Internet. The router configuration reads the address and redirects the information to the correct destination. The router usually seeks the least crowded pathway to prevent overload on particular lines on the Internet.

Search engine A computer program that has the capability of searching a specified group of pages on the WWW. The user gives the engine a word or group of words (search string) and it goes through its database to find those sites containing the search string.

Search string   The word or phrase that the user offers a search engine. In computerese a word is a "string of alphanumeric characters" and that is what the search engine computer will search for. Search strings may use Boolean terms to describe the inclusions or exclusions to the search.

Server   A computer connected to the Internet that will provide (serve) copies of files resident in its storage space and send them over the Internet on demand.

Shareware   Applications distributed on the Internet without immediate payment. Often these are a scaled-down version of a program you may want to buy but would like to try first. Sometimes the shareware program has full features but will only run for a few days.

Site or Web site   A group of pages posted and linked with a common purpose; usually this is the product of a single person, family, institution, or commercial entity.

Site map   A section of a Web site that explains the structure of the site and usually gives links to virtually all the major subsections. You should be able to tell from a well-constructed site map whether the information you need is on the site and how to get to it.

Software   The program or set of instructions that the computer interprets to run an application. Each instruction is extremely simple but the result of all the combined instructions gives rise to the complexity and power of the applications. The obverse is that a bug in the software can cause devastating consequences and is often very difficult to find (see Hardware).

SPAM   Unwanted junk messages sent to your e-mail address, usually advertising something or offering an unwanted service. The name derives from the Monty Python song. To SPAM is to send such messages broadcast to your mailing list or to the people in your address book and should be avoided.

Splash page   A page designed to attract attention with graphics or animated graphics and very little else. They usually have a link to the home page of the site. Splash pages are there because they are very attractive to search engines. A page with very little text scores very highly in the algorithm search engines use to rate pages assembled in response to a search request.

Surfing   Jumping from page to page on the World Wide Web pursuing links. May have pejorative connotations because the activity is superficial, or positive ones because it is fun. Surfing is probably the best way to get a feel for the immensity, the stunning variety, and the variable quality of the WWW.

Tags   The instructions embedded in an HTML file that determine the way the text of the file is displayed. These tags typically take the form ⟨tag⟩ for the beginning of the instruction and ⟨/tag⟩ for the end.

TCP/IP   Transmission control protocol / Internet protocol. The protocol that allows e-mail to be broken up into small packets, routed through many computers, and reassembled at the destination e-mail address.

Telnet   The software that allows a dialup connection between computers.

TIFF file   Tagged image format file. This uncompressed file is the standard image file used for printing.

Trojan   A malicious program similar to a virus that is designed to enable a hacker to access your computer files. The Trojan may create a "backdoor" into your computer and then send the details back to the hacker.

URL   Universal resource locator. The address of a Web page. For example, the URL of the Arthroscopy Association is **http://www.aana.org.** This is actually a number such as 881.234.111.452. The text is easier to remember, but each site is actually assigned a number or address on the Internet. When you register a new domain name, this is assigned a number and is activated by the service provider where you have the Web site.

Virus   A malicious program spread via the Internet or by exchanging infected files. The program is usually in machine language (and so is platform-specific). Currently the most common form of virus is one that is spread by e-mail messages. If you open an infected message, the virus code (instructions) is written into memory on your computer. When the instructions are activated they usually lead to attempts to replicate the code and spread it from your computer to others and the "payload," the damage the computer will do to your system (see Trojan).

Web	See Internet.
Webmaster	The individual who designs, oversees, and usually posts the pages on a site. He or she is not necessarily a major contributor of content to the site but has expertise in layout, HTML, and Web site management.
Web page	See Page.
Web site	See Site.
Window	A display technique supported by your computer's OS whereby output from an individual application is displayed in its own segment of your computer's monitor screen. Windows can be maximized to take up all the screen, resized to the shape and size you want, or minimized to an icon. Clicking on a particular window or double clicking on an icon makes that program the active one. Microsoft WINDOWS™ is the operating system for most PCs.
Wizard	An interactive program that assists you in undertaking certain actions in a specific program. They are used for complex parts of the application such as setup and registration.
WWW	World Wide Web. The collection of Web pages posted on the Internet that are viewed with a browser.
WYSIWYG	What you see is what you get. This is a term used for HTML editors meaning that the typing format you see on screen is the same format that will appear on the HTML page. This is not always the case and depends on the browser that is used.
Zip disc	A popular hardware add-on to computers without enough memory, for backup or for transferring substantial amounts of information between computers. Zip discs hold 100 megabytes of data. They are to some extent superseded by rewritable CD-ROMs.
ZIP file	This is a compressed file in WINDOWS™ that is used to compress documents sent by e-mail.

Index